The

Amino Acid

Report

Maximize the power of vegetarian protein

LINDA LAZARIDES

School of Modern Naturopathy

Other works by Linda Lazarides

Principles of Nutritional Therapy
The Nutritional Health Bible
The Waterfall Diet
Gourmet Nutritional Therapy Cookbook
A Textbook of Modern Naturopathy
Linda's Flat Stomach Secrets
The Big Healthy Soup Diet
Easy Water Retention Diet

About the Author

Linda Lazarides is one of Britain's most respected natural health experts, author of eight books, founder of the British Association for Nutritional Therapy, and Principal of the School of Modern Naturopathy.

2nd Edition (revised and expanded)
©Linda Lazarides 2016
www.naturostudy.org

ISBN-13: 978-1533377326
ISBN-10: 1533377324

Published in the United Kingdom.

Linda Lazarides asserts the moral right
to be identified as the author of this work.

Disclaimer

Every effort has been made to ensure accuracy, but the information presented herein is not intended as a substitute for medical advice. The book is sold on the understanding that the publisher and author are not liable for any misconception or misuse of the information provided and shall have neither liability nor responsibility to any person or entity with respect to any loss, damage or injury caused or alleged to be caused directly or indirectly by the said information.

CONTENTS

Part I

Protein Power

Part II

The Amino Acids

Appendix I

PART I

Protein Power

I. What is Protein?

Most of the human body consists of protein in different forms: muscles, hormones, enzymes, skin, hair, organs and, for bones, the fabric to which calcium clings. The type of protein simply depends on how its building blocks, the amino acids, are organized and linked together.

The amino acids are made from different arrangements of carbon, oxygen, hydrogen and nitrogen. Short sequences of amino acids are known as 'peptides', longer ones as 'polypeptides'. They are held together with bonds known as peptide bonds. Polypeptides can be several hundred amino acids long and when combined together can form thousands of different proteins.

Groups of amino acids

Apart from being used to make proteins in the body, most amino acids have various other tasks. The following work together:

- Branched chain amino acids: leucine, isoleucine, valine, important for muscles.
- Sulphur amino acids: cysteine, glutathione, taurine, methionine, important for detoxification.
- Urea cycle amino acids: arginine, citrulline, ornithine, important for removing ammonia.
- Glucogenic amino acids: primarily alanine, cysteine, glycine, serine, threonine, can be directly used to make glucose which the body can turn into energy.

Isomers

Amino acids can occur in two isomer forms (arrangements) known as the 'D' and 'L' forms. This is why you will often see them described as L-tryptophan or L-tyrosine for instance. The 'D' form of amino acids is not usually found in nature and, with the exception of D-phenylalanine, is not normally utilizable by the human body.

Some amino acids are more essential than others

The amino acids in the table below are often referred to as 'essential'. This can be misleading, since all amino acids are essential. In fact these are the amino acids which the body cannot manufacture. They are called essential because it is essential to get them from your food.

What happens to protein when you eat it?

Protein in your food is broken down by your digestive juices into peptides and then into individual amino acids. Amino acids are able to cross through the walls of your intestines into your bloodstream. From here they are picked up and 'knitted' into different types of protein. After eating a meal high in protein, your body works overtime to manufacture proteins, especially those for the liver and muscles, and serum albumin, a type of blood protein.

Essential Amino Acids

- Histidine
- Isoleucine
- Leucine
- Lysine
- Methionine
- Phenylalanine
- Threonine
- Tryptophan
- Valine

Any excess amino acids which cannot be used to make protein are broken down ready to be converted to glucose or to acetyl-CoA for making energy. They can also be stored as glycogen (stored carbohydate) and triglyceride (stored fat).

As the absorption of amino acids from your intestine begins to slow down after a meal, the synthesis of albumin and muscle protein also slows. If glycogen stores are used up before you eat again, your muscles begin to release amino acids as fuel for energy production. This is why when you go on a low-calorie diet you lose lean tissue or muscle at the same time as body fat. But if you stay on a low-calorie diet for a long time, your metabolism will eventually slow down in order to reduce lean tissue loss.

As amino acids are broken down, ammonia is formed. This is a toxin and must be converted by the liver to urea which can be excreted in the urine. The liver needs magnesium and several other nutrients to do this. If there is a shortage of these nutrients, ammonia builds up and depletes supplies of alpha-ketoglutarate, which is needed by the important Krebs cycle, a sequence of steps in which products made from glucose are turned into energy. If the Krebs cycle does not work well, fatigue and weakness occur. Excess ammonia also causes headaches, lethargy, irritability, and allergy-like reactions when high-protein foods are eaten.

Protein deficiency

Severe protein deficiency (mainly seen in developing countries) is known as kwashiorkor. Children need more protein than adults, and if they do not get enough their growth will be affected. Other effects of protein deficiency include impairment of digestion, fluid retention (due to the liver's failure to synthesize serum albumin), muscle wasting and anaemia.

Vegetarians

High-protein foods include meat, fish, eggs and other animal products, soy products, beans, lentils, nuts and seeds. Vegetable proteins are often low in some amino acids. These are known as the 'limiting' amino acids, for instance lysine in grains and seeds, and methionine in pulses (legumes) and soy products. This has given rise to a concept that vegans, who eat only plant foods, should carefully combine their foods to ensure that each meal provides a good balance of all the essential amino acids. In fact, several human studies now show that this is not necessary, at least in healthy volunteers eating rice-based diets, provided that the diets yield enough calories. When compared with those eating both rice and chicken, volunteers eating diets in which the protein was derived virtually only from rice, showed no significant difference in nitrogen balance, indicating that their protein intake was sufficient. Rice as the sole source of their protein still provided between 1.5 and 4.5 times the WHO recommended amounts of all the essential amino acids.

The American Dietetic Association now confirms that, because amino acids obtained from food can combine with amino acids made in the body, it is not necessary for vegans or vegetarians to combine protein foods at each meal. The ADA furthermore states that soy protein concentrate has been shown to be nutritionally equivalent in protein value to proteins of animal origin and so can serve as the sole source of protein intake if desired.

Since this statement, there has been growing evidence that the excessive consumption of soy protein concentrate—a highly processed product—could interfere with the function of the thyroid gland and could cause raised oestrogen levels in children. Obtaining protein from varied sources is probably the most sensible option.

Minimum protein requirements

The adult minimum protein requirement is 45 grams a day for women and 55 grams a day for men. A highly excessive protein intake can lead to an over-acid condition of the body, excessive ammonia levels, and—by increasing calcium excretion—osteoporosis.

Amino acid supplements

Some authorities have made statements that amino acid supplementation is pointless because most people in the western world already eat too much protein. In fact this fails to take account of individual biochemistry and possible errors of metabolism. Some people may be less capable than others of synthesizing 'non-essential' amino acids and would therefore benefit from supplementation, especially if they do not regularly consume animal products in their diet. Some individuals whose digestive ability is in a weakened state—perhaps due to illness or to age-related lack of adequate stomach acidity—may also need amino acid supplements.

The *Amino Acid Report* gives details of many research studies where amino acid supplements have proved beneficial for diseases that modern medical science is powerless to reverse. These include Alzheimer's disease, mental illness, chronic fatigue syndrome, herpes virus infections and gallbladder disease.

Now that detailed figures for amino acids in food have recently become available, healthy people are more easily able to adjust their amino acid balance using food. The *Amino Acid Report* will help you compare the amino acid content of many vegetarian foods, and dispels the myth that you have to eat meat to get enough protein.

Foods selected for inclusion in the tables

We attempted to provide a representative sample of vegetarian health foods. A selection of meat and fish foods has also been included for comparison purposes.

The cooked or uncooked, peeled or unpeeled status of the foods was chosen with a view to ease of comparison. For instance, although due to loss of water content protein becomes more concentrated in meat once it is cooked, its weight is then normally unknown to the cook, and it cannot then be compared with, say, 100 grams of roasted peanuts or a pound of potatoes, which weigh roughly the same once boiled. This is why for meat and fish the figures are for the raw state, while for other foods the figures are for states in which they are commonly eaten.

II. Aminos and detoxification

Every year after Christmas, a crop of articles usually appears in the media, encouraging us to go on a 'detox diet' to clear out our system after a season of self-indulgence. The diets are mostly based on raw fruit and vegetables, with herbal teas to replace caffeine, and strict abstinence from alcohol. Sometimes juices such as lemon or apple juice are added. More eccentric versions—also known as fasts—may call for eating only one or two foods, or for drinking just one type of juice or herbal tea.

The basic detox diet originally stems from traditional naturopathy—a natural medicine philosophy which was developed at the end of the 19th Century by doctors who were concerned at the toxicity of the conventional medicines—including mercury and arsenic—of the day. Naturopathic medicine was also known as 'nature cure', since it was believed to work by stimulating the body's own ability to heal itself. Naturopathic diets were thought not just to nourish the body, but to 'cleanse' it internally, 'purify the blood' and remove the 'toxins' which were causing the illness.

There is no doubt that naturopathic diets can have excellent results. Dr Max Gerson, who in the 1930s used naturopathic philosophy to pioneer the Gerson anti-cancer diet, had many remarkable successes, and the Gerson clinic, now based in Mexico, continues to help many cancer patients who have been failed by conventional treatments.

Some of the problems which modern conventional doctors have with believing in the value of naturopathic diets are:

- What are these 'toxins' which are supposed to cause illness?
- How is a diet of raw fruit and vegetables supposed to get rid of them?
- Such diets can be very low in calories, and may cause weakness, loss of vitality and weight loss. Some sick people can be made worse from this rather than better.

Cleansing effects or just low-calorie effects?

Adhering to a naturopathic cleansing diet often results in headaches, fatigue and weakness, even in healthy people. Naturopathic practitioners may attribute these symptoms to 'the toxins coming out', but this is not necessarily true. Headaches are the usual symptom of caffeine withdrawal. You are just as likely to get them simply by giving up tea and coffee without making any other changes to your diet. You can also get headaches from any low-calorie diet if you have a tendency to develop low blood sugar. Low-calorie diets also cause weakness and fatigue because they do not provide the amount of energy to which your body is accustomed, and so force you to begin breaking down your own body fat and body protein and muscle to get enough fuel for your daily energy needs.

Some toxins will inevitably be released from body fat when it is used for fuel. These are fat-soluble toxins which the body has not been able to excrete. They have been stored in your body fat to keep them out of harm's way. The pesticide DDT, banned in the 1970s because it caused widespread contamination, is a typical example of the type of toxin that can still be found in human body fat in all parts of the world today. If you remain on any low-calorie diet for several weeks, quantities of such toxins will probably be released from storage into your bloodstream. As they circulate around your body they can make you feel quite tired and ill, and it is essential that your liver—your organ of detoxification—should be properly nourished to deal with them.

After completing a detox or cleansing diet, people often say they feel less sluggish, and more alert and energetic. There can be several reasons for this:

- Overloading your digestive system with food (especially fatty, sugary food) uses up a great deal of energy and is likely to make you feel mentally and physically lethargic. Excess saturated fat stresses your liver, and excess sugary food plays havoc with your balance of insulin and other hormones. Reducing the load will naturally help you feel better.
- Tea, coffee and alcoholic drinks are often the only drinks consumed by many people. Because all three are diuretics (making us urinate more) they can cause chronic dehydration. Replacing them with water, fruit juices and herbal teas can quickly improve hydration and so boost energy and vitality.
- For most of the year most people's diets are very low in fruit and vegetables—the foods your body really craves. On a detox diet, your body is glad to get some real food.
- Detox diets make the body more alkaline. An acid residue is left in our tissues when our habitual diet is

too high in fat and protein. The more over-acidic your body, the less oxygen can get to your tissues and so the more prone to disease they can become. Eating fruit and vegetables (even sour ones) helps to reduce this acidity since your body metabolizes them (breaks them down) to an alkaline residue.

So if we cannot really be sure whether detox diets are in fact capable of removing toxins, should we perhaps look at the science to see whether there is research that makes a contribution to the subject of natural detoxification?

The liver: your organ of detoxification

In recent years, scientists have had a great deal to say about detoxification. As scientific knowledge about the workings of the body grows, the concept of toxins as a cause of disease is becoming more and more plausible. We now know that what the early naturopaths referred to as 'toxins' fall into three basic categories:

- *Xenobiotics*, which means substances foreign to the body, such as lead, mercury, drugs, pesticides and other chemical pollutants,
- *Metabolic wastes*: substances such as ammonia and aldehydes, produced in the course of the body's normal metabolism,
- *Endotoxins*: waste matter produced by the bacteria which normally live in our intestines. These toxins can be absorbed from the intestines into our bloodstream.

The removal of these from the body depends on four main organs:

- The liver, which processes toxins and prepares them for excretion,

- The intestines, which eliminate fat-soluble toxins in the stools,
- The kidneys, which extract water-soluble toxins from the blood,
- The skin, which excretes a variety of toxins in the sweat.

The lungs can expel mucus laden with wastes that come from quite deep within the tissues. Even hair and fingernails can help the body to excrete toxins. Toxic metals such as lead, mercury and arsenic can be found in the structure of the hair and in finger- and toenails, where they have been deposited out of harm's way.

So perhaps we can now begin to understand the problem which scientists and doctors have with the concept that food itself can detoxify you. The right foods (those rich in dietary fibre) can certainly help your intestines to expel toxins and wastes found in your stools. Some foods and herbs or spices, such as dandelion, beetroot and turmeric, can help to speed up the drainage of neutralized toxins and wastes from your liver into your gall-bladder, which releases them into your intestines. Foods such as celery seeds, fennel seeds or caraway seeds can make you urinate more. But in the end it is your organs, not your food, which detoxify you.

Your liver does its job by producing thousands of enzymes which help to break down the many toxins and waste products that challenge it daily. To produce these enzymes, it needs a steady supply of many different vitamins, minerals, antioxidant nutrients and amino acids. Amino acids are some of the most vital of liver nutrients, but they are in short supply in most naturopathic detox diets. This may not be a problem in the short term, provided that your liver enzymes are working well. But for individuals such as Teresa, whose case history is described below, it could make their health problems worse.

Teresa: a case of toxic overload

Teresa was a commercial artist who in the early part of her career had to use many chemicals now known to be hazardous to health. After a bout of ill health, involving several years of prescription medicines followed by an operation, Teresa's health broke down completely, and she was diagnosed with chronic fatigue syndrome, also known as ME. Disillusioned with conventional medicine, Teresa decided to consult a naturopath, who placed her on a 'blood purifying diet' of raw food and fresh vegetable juices. Teresa felt better in some ways—clearer-headed and 'lighter', but her fatigue did not improve, and the more weight she lost on the diet, the worse grew her physical weakness. By the time Teresa needed 15 hours of sleep a day and had to give up work, she gave up consulting the naturopath, and asked her doctor to refer her to a doctor of environmental medicine, for assessment of her level of toxins and liver function.

Traces of carbon tetrachloride and other toxic chemicals were found in Teresa's body tissues, and her liver function was only one third of normal. Her environmental medicine practitioner told her that she was not eating enough protein to make the liver enzymes she needed, and asked her to eat chicken, fish, nuts and sunflower seeds, plus rice, fruit and cooked vegetables rather than raw. He prescribed supplements of the amino acids n-acetyl cysteine and taurine, milk thistle herbal extract to repair her liver cells, and lipoic acid to help boost glutathione levels. Within three months, Teresa's liver enzymes were working much more normally, and, although it would be a long time before her body would recover from its slow poisoning, her health was no longer deteriorating.

Amino acids and detoxification

In the liver, toxins are combined or react with a variety of substances which help them to be broken down and turned into acids which can be more easily excreted. These substances include

- Oxygen
- Antioxidants
- Indoles from broccoli, brussels sprouts, cauliflower and cabbage
- Sulphate
- Acetyl groups
- Methyl groups
- Glucuronic acid
- Amino acids

The most important amino acids are

- **Cysteine**: helps to detoxify mercury, lead and arsenic, paracetamol (acetaminophen), steroids, contraceptive pill, aniline food dyes, terpenes, phenols and tyramine,
- **Glutathione**: helps to detoxify penicillin, tetracycline, petroleum products (including diesel smoke) toxic metals, bacterial toxins and alcohol,
- **Methionine**: helps to break down excess histamine and hormones and to detoxify phenols, sulphites, hypochlorites, morphine, paraquat, mercury, lead, arsenic and tin,

- **Glycine**: helps to detoxify phenols, aspirin, toluene, xylene, benzene, benzoate preservative, bile acids,
- **Taurine**: helps to detoxify chlorine compounds (including carbon tetrachloride) and to prevent the formation of toxic aldehydes, such as acetaldehyde.

Carnitine is also now thought to play a part in liver detoxification. Carnitine also reduces levels of lactic acid, which is formed in muscles (and makes them ache) when they are exercised without enough oxygen. Chronic fatigue sufferers often have high levels of lactic acid in their muscles, even when they have not been exercising.

Certain amino acids are also vital for the breakdown and excretion of ammonia, a toxin produced from protein. These include arginine, ornithine, aspartic acid, glutamic acid and glutamine.

Another type of metabolic toxin known as 'ketones', is formed when body fat is used for fuel (as when following any low-calorie diet). High ketone levels acidify the body. The amino acid alanine, found in nuts, seeds and oats, helps to prevent the formation of ketones, and carnitine helps to control ketone levels.

Fruit and vegetables supply many nutrients which help to neutralize a variety of toxins, especially the toxins which the liver has oxidized. But as you will see in Part II, they contain only small amounts of amino acids. Without the detoxifying amino acids mentioned above, many damaging toxins cannot be broken down *at all*. Dr Max Gerson recognized this, which is why his anti-cancer diet is low in protein only for a short time, just long enough to reduce the body's levels of acid residue. Bread made from sprouted grains is allowed on the Gerson diet, and after a few weeks cottage cheese can be added. Protein-rich sprouted seeds and raw liver juice were also a part of Gerson's original diet.

The verdict on detoxification?

If your aim is to alkalinize your body, reduce the amount of saturated fat clogging your liver, and give your digestive system a rest, then there is nothing better than a traditional 'nature cure' cleansing diet of fruit and vegetables together with potassium-rich fruit and vegetable juices. Beetroot juice helps to drain wastes from the liver and gall-bladder. Celery juice speeds up the removal of acids and is especially good for people with arthritis, who are often over-acidic. Broccoli or cabbage juice can provide support for some important liver enzymes.

Your cleansing diet does not have to be all-raw. If you have a chilly constitution, you may find that too much raw food does not suit you, and makes you feel tired and weak. In the Chinese, macrobiotic and Ayurvedic systems of medicine, it is generally recommended that those suffering from any form of weakness should eat only small amounts of raw or cold food. Vegetables are also easier to digest when cooked, since heat breaks down the tough cellulose walls of plant cells.

The more meat, fish and dairy products you have eaten in the recent past, the higher will be the acid residues in your body. No-one has conducted research to find out exactly how long it takes to reduce these residues with a cleansing diet, but the chances are that the longer you go without eating sufficient protein to fulfil your needs for detoxifying amino acids, the more stressed your liver could become. You do not need to go to extremes, and you certainly do not need to eat meat, fish or dairy products to get enough amino acids. As you will see in Part II, nuts, beans, sunflower seeds and many grains are excellent sources of all the essential amino acids, and are often superior to animal products in protein content.

Some of the diseases thought to be linked to a toxic overload and overstressed liver include Parkinson's disease, motor neurone disease, Alzheimer's disease, multiple sclerosis and chronic fatigue syndrome.

Meal Plan for Detoxification

Breakfast

Mix medium or fine-ground gluten-free oatmeal with sunflower seeds and dried fruit, and soak overnight in enough water to make a porridge-like consistency. Do not refrigerate. In the morning, stir the mixture, check the consistency and add a little more water if necessary before serving.

Lunch

Mix cooked brown rice with finely chopped raw vegetables (e.g. carrots, spring onion (scallion) red and green peppers, celery). Flavour with pepper, herbs, lemon juice and a little extra virgin olive oil. Serve with cottage cheese or soft goat's cheese flavoured with herbs or garlic, plus home made fresh vegetable and lentil soup or miso soup. Do not overload your stomach. Follow with fresh fruit (orange, apple, pear, banana etc.).

Dinner

Avocado followed by cooked beans or lentils, braised with potatoes, onion and broccoli, cabbage, cauliflower or brussels sprouts plus any other vegetables to taste. Serve with a salad of fresh beetroot (beets), radish and grated carrot. Follow with stewed apples (retain the peel) with ground almonds and raisins. Do not overload your stomach.

Drinks

Spice tea, fennel, peppermint or ginger tea (tea bags are available for all these). Fresh juices made from any combination of beetroot, celery, broccoli, carrot or radish.

Snacks

Peanuts, fresh or roasted without oil and salt. Other fresh nuts. Fresh fruit. Organic dried fruit.

\Miso soup and spice tea bags can be found in health food stores and larger supermarkets.

III. Fighting fatigue

Chronic fatigue syndrome is also known as CFS or ME (myalgic encephalomyelitis). People who suffer from it feel exhausted all the time, even when they have not done anything physically demanding. They may need to sleep 10 or more hours a day, yet still feel unrefreshed in the morning. It is quite common for CFS sufferers to go straight to bed after work, if they are able to work at all. Some are house-bound, too weak to go for a walk or even for a car ride. Those with very severe chronic fatigue cannot even get out of bed, and may be conscious for only a few hours a day.

Chronic fatigue sufferers generally have a variety of other symptoms, which vary from person to person. Muscle pain (sometimes known as fibromyalgia) is the most common. It is like the ache you get in your muscles when you have over-exercised them. The difference is that a CFS sufferer has this pain all the time, even without having exercised. Also common are headaches and 'brain fatigue'—a frightening loss of the ability to concentrate on anything and get your head round any but the simplest thoughts. Causes of chronic fatigue include

- The lingering effects of viruses such as the Epstein-Barr virus, a member of the herpes virus family which causes glandular fever (infectious mononucleosis)
- A toxic overload, leading to symptoms upon exposure to small amounts of chemicals such as perfumes, air

fresheners, exhaust fumes, cleaning fluids or food additives
- Nutritional deficiencies
- Food intolerances
- Dysbiosis: a toxic condition of the intestines caused by overgrowths of bacteria and fungi, and often brought on by taking antibiotics. The bacterial toxins overload the liver, and can themselves cause headaches and severe fatigue.

Several amino acids can play a part in helping the body to combat chronic fatigue syndrome.

Glutathione and lysine

As you will see in Part II, low levels of glutathione seem to promote the growth of viruses. Chronic fatigue expert Dr Paul Cheney says that by raising glutathione levels you can stop almost any virus from replicating. Since many chronic fatigue sufferers seem at some time to have been infected with the Epstein-Barr virus, it makes sense to follow the advice given in Part II for maximizing glutathione levels in this condition.

On the other hand the amino acid arginine is thought to encourage the growth of viruses belonging—as Epstein-Barr does—to the herpes virus family. The best way to minimize the effects of arginine is to avoid foods such as gelatine and nuts with a high arginine to lysine ratio, and to take lysine supplements. You can read more about this in the section on lysine.

Carnitine and methionine

Carnitine is known to make muscles more efficient when exercising, and can reduce the amount of lactic acid produced when exercising. Lactic acid is responsible for post-exercise muscle ache and probably also for much of the muscle ache experienced by CFS sufferers. In a research study carried out on 30 CFS sufferers, carnitine was able to help 12 out of 18 of their symptoms within four to eight weeks.

Researchers have reported in the Scandinavian Journal of Rheumatology that methionine can also be used as a treatment for fibromyalgia, which is the name given to the muscle pain associated with chronic fatigue syndrome. No-one is sure why methionine has this effect, and some other researchers have not managed to get the same results. It was first attributed to methionine's role in making the body's natural pain-killers, known as enkephalins and endorphins, but this theory now seems to be disputed.

Branched-chain amino acids

An interesting new theory about the excessive drowsiness associated with chronic fatigue syndrome has recently appeared. Most of the symptoms sufferered by people with chronic fatigue are those which would normally be connected with over-exertion. Chronic fatigue sufferers are in fact constantly over-exerting themselves simply by normal day-to-day living. Their energy production capacity is so limited that it is depleted by extremely small amounts of activity.

One of the effects of normal over-exertion is the depletion within the muscles of the branched-chain amino acids leucine, isoleucine and valine, which are used for fuel. These amino acids compete with tryptophan for entry into the brain, which means that when they are depleted, tryptophan is able to enter the brain in larger than normal amounts.

Once tryptophan enters the brain, it is turned into a neurotransmitter (brain chemical) known as serotonin, which causes drowsiness and induces sleep. The more tryptophan is allowed to enter the brain, the more serotonin is produced.

Research badly needs to be carried out to measure levels of branched-chain amino acids in chronic fatigue sufferers, and to assess whether supplementation with leucine, isoleucine and valine can help to prevent excessive serotonin production. If so, it may be part of the answer to reducing drowsiness and excessive sleeping in chronic fatigue syndrome. Meanwhile, it is important for people with CFS to avoid consuming sugary food, since this aids the uptake of tryptophan into the brain and reduces levels of tyrosine, needed to make mood-elevating, anti-fatigue adrenal hormones.

Meal plan for chronic fatigue syndrome

Can also be used by people with herpes

Breakfast

Grilled (broiled) avocado and goat's cheese. Grilled herring if you are not vegetarian. Warm stewed fruit and sheep's milk yoghurt. (Many people with CFS are intolerant to cow's milk).

Lunch

Brown rice baked with ginger, cloves and other spices, finely chopped vegetables and tofu. Serve with stewed mung beans flavoured with onions and miso. Serve with a salad dressed with extra-virgin olive oil and chopped raw garlic, which both help to combat bacteria and fungi in the intestines. Follow with fresh fruit.

Dinner

Grilled or steamed fish, (use goat's cheese or tofu instead if you are vegetarian) potatoes and broccoli, cabbage, cauliflower or brussels sprouts. Include mushrooms if you are not allergic to them. Make a sauce with extra-virgin olive oil and chopped raw garlic, both of which help to combat bacteria and fungi in the intestines. Follow with baked fruit and sheep's milk yoghurt.

Drinks

Beetroot (beet) juice, spice tea, chamomile tea, ginger tea.

Snacks

Warm food, e.g. leftovers, baked beans, stewed fruit and yoghurt, vegetable and bean or lentil soup, warm butterbeans (lima beans) in a dressing of extra virgin olive oil, chopped spring onion, garlic and herbs. You can add canned fish if you are not vegetarian.

Spice tea bags and miso are available from health food stores.

IV. Heart protection

What most people refer to as heart disease is not actually a disease of the heart at all, but of the coronary arteries which supply your heart muscle with blood. Cholesterol deposits on the walls of these narrow arteries can eventually reduce the blood supply, leaving your heart short of oxygen. If the arteries become narrow enough, angina pain occurs due to the lack of oxygen whenever your heart is made to beat faster. Angina tends to get worse and to come on more easily as the clogging of the arteries progresses. Complete oxygen starvation, as when a small clot lodges in the already narrowed artery, is experienced as a heart attack or cardiac arrest—the heart stops functioning completely. Whether or not it starts up again depends on how soon the flow of blood through the heart is able to resume. If the heart tissue remains for too long without oxygen, too much of it will have died for the heart to resume beating.

After a heart attack, damage to your heart tissue often leads to abnormalities in your heart's structure and a reduced efficiency. As your heart struggles to keep up with its workload, it may in time start to fail—its pumping action cannot get blood around your body fast enough to keep all your organs supplied with enough oxygen and nutrients. This condition is known as congestive heart failure (CHF). The heart will often become enlarged as it attempts to work harder, and water retention can be a big problem as the kidneys fail to get the stimulation they need for working efficiently.

CHF can also develop without any previous damage to your heart, if your heart's workload becomes abnormally large for too long. Severe anaemia, for example, when the red blood cells are not able to absorb enough oxygen from the lungs, forces the heart to pump much harder as it attempts to get the blood around to the lungs again as quickly as possible. Other conditions which can damage the heart or increase its workload and so possibly lead to enlarged heart and CHF include:

- Alcoholism
- Severe vitamin B1 deficiency
- Untreated high blood pressure
- Thyroid abnormalities
- The lung diseases emphysema, asthma and chronic bronchitis
- Severe water retention
- Severe overweight.

Modern research shows that three amino acids can be used directly to combat heart disease.

Arginine, carnitine and taurine

Intensive research is being carried out into nitric oxide, a substance made from the amino acid arginine, which helps to relax and dilate blood vessels. By increasing amounts of nitric oxide, arginine-rich diets can help to control blood pressure and other problems associated with narrowing of the arteries, including angina and male erectile dysfunction.

Carnitine's ability to help the body use fat for energy production seems to be especially beneficial for the heart.

Carnitine also seems to be able to improve blood flow through the heart. Studies have shown that carnitine supplements can reduce angina, reduce the tendency to develop CHF after a heart attack, and improve the symptoms and extend the life span of people with CHF.

Taurine is the most abundant amino acid in the heart muscle, where it helps to balance mineral levels and stabilize the electrical activity. The heartbeat relies on electrical impulses and taurine is of great importance in helping to keep the heart beating normally. Taurine supplements have been successfully used to:

- Reduce abnormal heart rhythms caused by adrenaline (epinephrine in the U.S.)
- Encourage the excretion of sodium and excess fluid in CHF
- Improve the symptoms and extend the life span of people with CHF.

Homocysteine

Homocysteine is a toxic amino acid which has been linked with heart and artery disease, Alzheimer's disease, kidney disease and osteoporosis. As part of a normal process, it is formed within the body from the amino acids cysteine and methionine. It should be quickly broken down and rendered harmless by two enzymes, but a few individuals have a genetic defect which requires extra large amounts of B vitamins to support these enzymes, especially when cysteine or methionine consumption is high. Without the extra vitamins (vitamins B6, B12, folic acid and betaine), homocysteine levels in the blood can rise, causing many abnormalities including high cholesterol levels.

As well as the above-mentioned health problems, high homocysteine levels are an indicator of poor 'methylation'—a process which is required as part of liver detoxification, and involves the amino acid methionine and the above-listed B vitamins. Symptoms of poor liver detoxification are many and varied, and include headaches and chronic fatigue.

It has recently been discovered that the kidneys are involved in removing homocysteine from the blood. While homocysteine levels cause high cholesterol and are generally a sign of inadequate vitamins B6, B12, folic acid and betaine, they are also found in people with failing kidney function or chronic kidney disease. If an individual is supplementing these vitamins and still has high homocysteine levels he or she may unknowingly have kidney disease. One of the main causes of kidney disease is high blood pressure, so measures to bring down blood pressure should be taken as soon as possible. It is also possible that homocysteine itself damages kidney function[1].

Glycation and AGEs

High levels of sugar in our blood are extremely destructive. Glycation occurs when sugar attaches itself to amino acids, forming AGEs (Advanced Glycation End Products). These products destroy proteins in the body by crosslinking them, and also induce free radical formation and chronic inflammation. They are found in particularly high levels in diabetics, due to the higher sugar levels in their blood, but they also rise in non-diabetics as they get older, after a lifetime of exposure to sugar. Consuming proteins browned at high temperatures—e.g. barbecued food—will also raise levels of AGEs.

AGEs reduce the regenerative ability of collagen, promoting wrinkles and sagging of the skin. They have recently been shown to play an important role in the development of atherosclerosis—the clogging of the arteries which leads to heart attacks.

Carnosine, a dipeptide combining two amino acids—histidine and beta-alanine, can inhibit glycation and cross-linking, and is considered to have excellent anti-ageing properties.

One of the harmful effects of AGEs is to reduce the sensitivity of insulin, which stops insulin from working effectively to remove sugar from the blood. Insulin sensitivity can be restored by supplementation with n-acetylcysteine.

Cloves and cinnamon are the leading protective spices against AGEs, due to their phenol content. Phenols are compounds found in many plants, and have antioxidant properties. The total phenol content of cloves is 30 percent of its dry weight, which is much higher than blueberries, a food known for its content of antioxidants and phenols. The higher the phenol content of a food, the stronger its ability to block AGE formation.

References

1. Xie D, Yuan Y et al. Hyperhomocysteinemia predicts renal function decline: a prospective study in hypertensive adults. *Scientific Reports* 2015;5:16268.

Meal plan for a healthy heart

Breakfast

Porridge made with oats, nut or soy milk and liberal amounts of chopped Brazil nuts. Sweeten only with raisins.

Lunch

Mix cooked brown rice with finely chopped raw vegetables (e.g. carrots, spring onion (scallion) red and green peppers, celery). Flavour with pepper, herbs, lemon juice and extra virgin olive oil. Serve with canned fish or cottage cheese or soft goat's cheese flavoured with herbs or garlic, plus home made fresh vegetable and lentil soup or miso soup. You could also mix the vegetables with hummus and put in sandwiches made with wholemeal bread. Fresh fruit.

Dinner

Grilled or steamed salmon, mackerel or herring (use tofu or beans instead if you are vegetarian) plus potatoes and broccoli, cabbage, cauliflower or brussels sprouts. Moisten with a sauce made with extra virgin olive oil, onion, garlic and herbs. Serve with an organic green salad dressed with lemon juice and extra virgin olive oil. Follow with fresh fruit, which can be raw, baked or stewed. If you are not vegetarian, eat fresh fruit jelly (jello) regularly for arginine.

Drinks

Beet juice, spice tea, chamomile tea, fresh fruit juice.

Snacks

Peanuts, fresh or roasted without oil or salt. Brazil nuts, walnuts, almonds, hazelnuts etc. Oatcakes with almond butter, topped with all-fruit sugar-free jam. Fresh vegetable soup. Fresh fruit.

Miso soup and spice tea bags can be found in health food stores and larger supermarkets.

V. A youthful brain

One of the problems we fear most as we age is senility—the loss of our mental functions. This can begin in middle age with a decline in short-term memory—a reduction in your ability to recall recent events, telephone numbers, or where you put your car keys.

This ageing process does not necessarily have anything to do with the number of birthdays we have had. Certain factors can accelerate the ageing of those parts of our body which are responsible for memory. This deterioration can accumulate with age, but if the factors responsible can be prevented, there is no reason why we should not have as good a memory when we are 90 as we did when we were 30.

Three types of deterioration have so far been identified:

- Loss of nerve cells
- Damage to nerve cells
- Reduced production and increased breakdown of the important brain chemical acetylcholine.

The adrenal hormones adrenaline (also known as epinephrine), noradrenaline and dopamine are important for memory and concentration.

Arginine

Like most other types of cells, nerve cells need a rich supply of blood to bring them nutrients and oxygen. But cholesterol deposits in arteries as we get older lead to increasingly poor blood circulation. Because of its role in the production of nitric oxide, which relaxes blood vessels and so improves blood flow, the amino acid arginine has great potential as a treatment for age-related memory loss. In one study, in which elderly people were given 1.6 grams a day of supplementary arginine, their score for mental ability improved by more than 50 per cent in three months. They also showed more expressive faces and quicker responses. This improvement was lost when the arginine supplements were stopped. You can read more about this in the chapter on arginine.

Carnitine

Acetyl L-carnitine is the form best assimilated into the brain. Research shows that it has much potential for the treatment of Alzheimer's disease and geriatric depression. This ability is probably related to carnitine's ability to improve the circulation and to enhance the production of acetylcholine—the body's prime memory aid.

Taurine

In one study, 3-4 grams a day of taurine supplementation was found to reduce dementia in elderly people after several weeks. The reason for this effect is not clear. One theory is that because taurine helps to stimulate the production of hydrochloric acid by the stomach, these elderly people were able to digest and assimilate their food better, thus improving their body's ability to make a variety of hormones and neurotransmitters (substances which govern brain activity and nerve impulses). Taurine is also a powerful aid to liver detoxification, and may help to reduce levels of toxins which can damage nerve cells.

Tyrosine

Mental ability, alertness and concentration are highly dependent on the adrenal hormones adrenaline (epinephrine), noradrenaline and dopamine. These in turn are made from the amino acid tyrosine. We are not aware of any studies using tyrosine supplements against age-related mental decline, but the US Military has for some years conducted studies assessing the effects of tyrosine supplements on cadets subjected to demanding military combat training courses. Under these conditions, tyrosine seems to be able to reduce blood pressure, and to reduce the effects of stress and fatigue on the ability to perform mental tasks. More about this in the chapter on tyrosine.

Serine

Phosphatidylserine (PS), which is a combination of fat with phosphate and the amino acid serine, is an important structural component of nerve cell membranes. The scientific community is becoming very interested in the potential for PS supplementation to help reverse age-related memory problems and the deterioration of mental ability. Several encouraging double-blind studies have so far been carried out. Functions measured include:
- Learning names and faces
- Recalling names and faces
- Facial recognition
- Telephone number recall
- Misplaced objects recall
- Ability to concentrate while reading

- Recall of details of events from the previous day or the past week
- Word acquisition and recall.

Individuals treated with PS supplements experienced significant improvements in these functions, in some cases reversing their mental decline by the equivalent of up to 12 years. Those worst affected often showed the most improvement.

PS appears to work through its role in the conduction of the nerve impulse, the accumulation, storage and release of neurotransmitters (substances which regulate the nerve impulses), and the receptor sites on cell surfaces.

Methionine

One of the body's uses for the amino acid methionine is to make choline, a substance which is needed to synthesize the important memory neurotransmitter acetylcholine. Research using methionine, and especially s-adenosyl methionine supplementation against Alzheimer's disease is showing encouraging results.

Green tea

Green tea has a highly protective effect on brain cells. Scientists have used it to combat both Parkinson's disease and Alzheimer's disease[1,2].

Glycation

As explained on page 31, glycation is a harmful reaction between sugar and protein in the body. One of the effects of glycation is chronic inflammation of a type that has been linked with Alzheimer's disease[3].

AGEs (Advanced Glycation End Products) accumulate in the brain with increasing age and are found in nerve fibre tangles and senile plaques in patients with Alzheimer's disease. Diabetic patients are at higher risk of developing Alzheimer's disease, and the brains of diabetic patients with Alzheimer's disease tend to show larger deposits of AGEs[4].

See pages 31-32 for items which can help to combat AGEs.

References

1. Mandel SA, Amit T et al. Simultaneous manipulation of multiple brain targets by green tea catechins: a potential neuroprotective strategy for Alzheimer and Parkinson diseases. CNS Neurosci Ther. 2008 Winter;14(4):352-65.
2. Zhao B. Natural antioxidants protect neurons in Alzheimer's disease and Parkinson's disease. Neurochem Res. 2009 Apr;34(4):630-8.
3. Walker D, Lue LF et al. Receptor for advanced glycation endproduct modulators: a new therapeutic target in Alzheimer's disease. ExpertOpin Investig Drugs. 2015 Mar;24(3):393-9.
4. (Semba RD, Nicklett EJ et al. Does Accumulation of Advanced Glycation End Products Contribute to the Aging Phenotype? The Journals of Gerontology Series A: Biological Sciences and Medical Sciences. 2010;65A (9):963-975.

Meal plan for a healthy brain

Breakfast

Porridge made with oats, nut or soy milk and liberal amounts of chopped Brazil nuts or sunflower seeds. No sugar. Sweeten with raisins.

Lunch

Mix cooked brown rice with finely chopped raw vegetables (e.g. carrots, spring onion (scallion) red and green peppers, celery). Flavour with pepper, herbs, lemon juice and a little extra virgin olive oil. Serve with canned fish, cottage cheese or soft goat's cheese flavoured with herbs or garlic, plus home made fresh vegetable and lentil soup or miso soup. You could also mix the vegetables with hummus and put in sandwiches made with wholemeal bread. Fresh fruit.

Dinner

Grilled or steamed salmon, mackerel or herring (use tofu or beans instead if you are vegetarian) plus potatoes and broccoli, cabbage, cauliflower or brussels sprouts. Moisten with a sauce made with extra virgin olive oil, onion, garlic and herbs. Serve with an organic green salad dressed with lemon juice and extra virgin olive oil. Follow with fresh fruit, especially dark blue or purple fruit, which can be raw, baked or stewed. If you are not vegetarian, eat fresh fruit jelly (jello) regularly for arginine.

Drinks

Beet juice, chamomile tea, fresh fruit juice, spice tea.

Snacks

Peanuts, fresh or roasted without oil or salt. Brazil nuts, walnuts, almonds, hazelnuts etc. Oatcakes with almond butter, topped with all-fruit blueberry or bilberry jam. Fresh vegetable soup. Fresh fruit.

Spice tea bags and miso are available from health food stores.

VI. Mental Health

Known together as the 'catecholamines', abnormal levels of the adrenal hormones dopamine, adrenaline and noradrenaline, all of which are made from the amino acid tyrosine, are especially thought to play a part in clinical depression and mania. Individuals with depression excrete reduced amounts of catecholamines in their urine. Individuals with mania, on the other hand, excrete increased amounts. Monoamine oxidase inhibitors—drugs used to treat depression—work by inhibiting an enzyme which breaks down catecholamines, thus allowing higher concentrations of the hormones to circulate in the body. The drug lithium, used to treat mania, is thought to work by reducing the release of noradrenaline from nerve terminals and enhancing its uptake.

This role of the catecholamines in mood may explain the successes gained in trials using supplements of their raw materials—the amino acids tyrosine and phenylalanine—against clinical depression. The amino acid L-tryptophan is now a fairly standard medical treatment for the agitated form of depression, which is related to a serotonin neurotransmitter imbalance rather than a catecholamine deficiency.

One use of methionine supplements in mental illness is to help the body break down excessive levels of histamine, a body chemical which is found in large amounts in some cases of schizophrenia, especially those associated with an agitated form of depression and suicidal tendencies. According to Dr Carl Pfeiffer, who pioneered this treatment, high histamine individuals are at higher risk of developing schizophrenia, and their symptoms can be controlled by reducing their histamine levels with large doses of methionine and calcium.

Supplements of s-adenosyl methionine have been found helpful against depression.

Other nutritional factors which can influence mental health are deficiencies of B vitamins (especially folic acid), zinc and selenium, blood sugar imbalances and heavy metal toxicity.

Meal plan for mental health

Breakfast

Porridge made with oats, milk and liberal amounts of chopped Brazil nuts and sunflower seeds. No sugar—sweeten with raisins. Avocado smoothie with milk and banana.

Lunch

Mix cooked brown rice with finely chopped raw vegetables (e.g. carrots, spring onion (scallion) red and green peppers, celery). Flavour with pepper, herbs, lemon juice and extra virgin olive oil. Serve with canned fish or cheese, plus home made fresh vegetable and lentil soup or miso soup. You could also mix the vegetables with hummus and put in sandwiches made with wholemeal bread. Fresh fruit, dried fruit, walnuts.

Dinner

Grilled or steamed salmon, mackerel or herring (use eggs, cheese, tofu or beans instead if you are vegetarian) plus potatoes and broccoli, cabbage, cauliflower or brussels sprouts. Moisten with a sauce made with extra virgin olive oil, onion, garlic and herbs. Serve with an organic green salad dressed with lemon juice and extra virgin olive oil. Follow with fresh fruit, which can be raw, baked or stewed.

Drinks

Mixed vegetable juice, spice tea, ginger tea, fresh fruit juice.

Snacks

Peanuts, fresh or roasted without oil or salt. Fruit yoghurt, cheese. Brazil nuts, sunflower seeds. Oatcakes with almond butter, topped with all-fruit sugar-free jam. Fresh vegetable soup. Avocados and fresh fruit.

Spice tea bags and miso are available from health food stores.

VII. Aminos for athletes

The two most outstanding uses of amino acids in sports are for
- Body building
- Endurance sports

Alanine

Together with L-histidine, alanine forms the dipeptide carnosine, found in large amounts in the muscles. By acting as a buffer—helping to reduce acidosis—carnosine increases the muscle fatigue threshold.

The International Society of Sports Nutrition (ISSN) has issued the following statements about the supplement beta-alanine:
- Four weeks of beta-alanine supplementation significantly augments muscle carnosine concentrations, thus acting as an intracellular pH buffer
- Daily supplementation with 4 to 6 g of beta-alanine for at least 2 to 4 weeks has been shown to improve exercise performance, especially in tasks 1 to 4 minutes in duration
- Beta-alanine attenuates neuromuscular fatigue, particularly in older individuals.

Arginine and ornithine

There is some evidence that supplements of these two amino acids may stimulate the release of growth hormone and insulin, and so increase muscle bulk. Dr Eric Braverman, author of *the Healing Nutrients Within*, suggests that ornithine is a better arginine supplement than arginine itself, because it enters the mitochondria (the energy-producing part of the cell) more readily than arginine. The body readily converts ornithine to arginine. Most scientists doubt that these two amino acids really can have a significant effect, because the research is scanty. Some researchers say that very large doses are necessary to achieve any effect at all, and others say that increases in lean body mass and strength can be achieved with just one gram a day of each amino acid.

Branched-chain amino acids

In any intensive athletic activity, especially endurance sports, carbohydrate stores can be quickly depleted. The branched-chain amino acids (which form part of muscle protein) are then used as fuel. Leucine can be used directly as an energy source. Valine can be converted to glucose. Isoleucine can be converted either to glucose or to ketones, both of which can be used as an energy source. Alanine and glutamate can also be converted to glucose. It is becoming recognized that supplementation with these amino acids helps to prevent the breakdown of body proteins and can significantly prolong energy in endurance sports.

Tryptophan

Strenuous physical exercise brings on discomfort and pain. The body's enkephalins and endorphins produced during exercise help us to tolerate this pain. In turn serotonin, produced from tryptophan, plays a part in regulating the enkephalins and endorphins. Research has shown that tryptophan supplements taken before intensive exercise can reduce the feeling of over-exertion, allowing athletes to extend their normal exercise tolerance by up to 50 per cent.

Tyrosine and methionine

These are the raw materials of the enkephalins and endorphins. Tyrosine is also needed to make the hormones adrenaline (ephinephine in the US), noradrenaline and dopamine. These are involved in alertness, concentration, and helping the body to find extra energy in stressful or competitive situations. Research is currently in progress by the US military authorities, using tyrosine supplements to counteract the stress and fatigue seen in sustained military operations consisting of continuous work periods exceeding 12 hours and often involving sleep loss.

Glutamine

Intensive exercise is highly stressful to the body, and is known to deplete the immune system, leading to a higher than normal rate of infections. Research has found that supplementation with the amino acid glutamine can reduce the rate of infections in athletes undergoing prolonged exhaustive exercise. This is because during periods of severe metabolic stress, the body's requirements for glutamine may exceed the ability to produce sufficient amounts. Glutamine supplementation has beneficial effects on nitrogen balance and muscle protein metabolism as well as immune status. Glutamine can be turned into glucose if needed for fuel.

Meal plan for athletes

Breakfast

Porridge made with milk and liberal amounts of chopped Brazil nuts and sunflower seeds. No sugar—sweeten with raisins. Avocado smoothie with milk and banana.

Lunch

Mix cooked brown rice with finely chopped raw vegetables (e.g. carrots, spring onion (scallion) red and green peppers, celery). Flavour with pepper, herbs, lemon juice and extra virgin olive oil. Serve with canned fish or cheese, plus home made fresh vegetable and lentil soup or miso soup. You could also put the ingredients in sandwiches made with wholemeal bread. Follow with fresh fruit, dried fruit and walnuts.

Dinner

Grilled or steamed salmon, mackerel or herring (use eggs, cheese, tofu or beans instead if you are vegetarian) plus potatoes and broccoli, cabbage, cauliflower or brussels sprouts. Moisten with a sauce made with extra virgin olive oil, onion, garlic and herbs. Serve with an organic green salad dressed with lemon juice and extra virgin olive oil. Follow with fresh fruit, which can be raw, baked or stewed. If you are not vegetarian, eat fresh fruit jelly (jello) for branched-chain amino acids and alanine.

Drinks

Celery juice, spice tea, ginger tea, fresh fruit juice.

Snacks

Peanuts, fresh or roasted without oil or salt. Fruit yoghurt, cheese. Brazil nuts, walnuts, almonds, hazelnuts etc. Oatcakes with almond butter, topped with all-fruit sugar-free jam. Fresh vegetable soup. Avocados and fresh fruit.

Spice tea bags and miso are available from health food stores.

PART II

The Amino Acids

Alanine

What does the body use alanine for?

- Helps to prevent ketosis
- Can be turned into glucose if necessary
- Can trigger the release of glucagon from the pancreas
- Inhibitory neurotransmitter
- Needed for the production of white blood cells
- Together with L-histidine, forms the anti-ageing dipeptide carnosine, found mostly in red meat.

What foods is it found in?

- Gelatine
- Meat, fish
- Sunflower seeds
- Almonds
- Peanuts
- Oats

Alanine is also made in the body from pyruvate (a substance involved in energy metabolism) and from the breakdown of DNA. With the aid of zinc it can be formed in the muscles from the peptide carnosine. Nitrogen from branched-chain amino acids in the muscles is used to form alanine and glutamine.

Useful information

Alanine is found in large amounts in the muscles. When released from the muscles it can be readily converted into glucose by the liver and so used as a source of energy.

Alanine and glutamine are the most important of the amino acids that help to keep up levels of glucose for the body to use as fuel. When carbohydrate stores are exhausted, large amounts of alanine and glutamine are released from the muscles and serve to shuttle nitrogen and carbon (derived from amino acids) to other tissues. This carbon can be converted to glucose by the liver and used to produce energy.

The metabolism of diabetics seems to use a great deal more alanine and glutamine for producing glucose than does the metabolism of healthy people[1] .

Glucagon is a hormone produced by the pancreas, which helps to raise blood sugar (glucose) levels when they drop too low. Alanine can stimulate the release of glucagon.

Neurotransmitters regulate the electrical impulses which pass along nerves. As an inhibitory neurotransmitter, alanine helps to control these impulses.

Alanine helps to prevent ketones from forming. Ketosis is a toxic condition resulting from excess ketones in the body. Ketones are produced when fat is used by the body as fuel because carbohydrate is not available. This situation occurs:

- During low-calorie diets
- After intensive exercise which uses up carbohydrate stores
- In diabetes.

Diabetics, who may have plenty of carbohydrate in their blood but cannot use it—quickly develop ketosis if their disease is not treated. The acetone odour which is noticed on the breath of someone in a diabetic coma is due to the large amount of ketones in the blood.

Lactate and pyruvate, which are produced in the muscles from glucose metabolism, can be converted to alanine. This alanine can then be converted back to glucose. This process is known as the glucose-alanine cycle, and can provide as much as 5 per cent of the total fuel needed during prolonged exercise.

Muscle endurance

After eight experienced resistance-trained men were given 30 days of beta-alanine supplementation at 4.8 g per day, no change was seen in testosterone concentrations but muscular endurance was significantly improved[2].

Body mass

After six weeks of supplementation with beta-alanine, forty-four women following a high intensity interval training programme were found to have increased body mass compared with controls[3].

High-intensity exercise

Beta-alanine supplementation has been shown to improve exercise performance metabolism in short-term, high-intensity efforts such as severe cycling, running 800 metres, and ski-ing. It results in a delay in the onset of muscular fatigue, and a facilitated recovery during repeated bouts of high-intensity exercise[4,5,6].

Elderly frailty

A nutritional supplement fortified with 800-1200 mg beta-alanine was shown to improve physical working capacity, muscle quality and function in men and women with an average age of 70 years[7].

Military activity

Recent studies in military personnel support the use of beta-alanine supplementation to enhance combat-specific performance. There appears to be most benefit for high-intensity activity lasting 60-300 seconds. There is also a small amount of evidence that beta-alanine supplementation may enhance cognitive function and promote resiliency during highly stressful situations[8].

SUPPLEMENTS

The use of beta-alanine supplementation has been exponentially growing in recent years. It is used by athletes competing in high-intensity track and field cycling, rowing, swimming events and other competitions.

The effects of supplementation with beta-alanine have been attributed to its ability to increase carnosine levels in the body. The supplements are available in powdered form as a pre–workout supplement. Doses used in research range from 2 to 6 grams per day. Higher doses only appear to be slightly more effective if the supplement is taken every day.

How safe are beta-alanine supplements?

The International Society of Sports Nutrition (ISSN) advises that beta-alanine supplementation of up to 6 grams per day currently appears to be safe in healthy individuals. The only reported side effect is paraesthesia (tingling), but this can be reduced by using divided doses (e.g. 1.5 grams, four times a day)[9].

Alanine content of common foods
in grams per 100g

Gelatine, dry	8.01
Tuna, skipjack, fresh, raw	1.33
Salmon, Atlantic, farmed, raw	1.20
Prawns, boiled	1.18
Chicken meat, raw	1.17
Beef, ground, extra-lean (approx. 21% fat)	1.16
Sunflower seeds, hulled	1.12
Pork, composite of various cuts, trimmed, raw	1.11
Herring, Atlantic, raw	1.09
Almonds, raw	1.00
Peanuts, dry roasted	0.94
Oats	0.88
Buckwheat flour, whole groat	0.71
Cheese, cheddar	0.70
Walnuts, raw	0.70
Eggs, hard-boiled	0.70
Cornmeal, whole-grain, yellow	0.61
Brazil nuts, raw	0.57
Wheat flour, whole-grain	0.49
Chick peas, boiled	0.38
Lentils, boiled	0.38
Tofu, raw, with calcium sulphate	0.77
Yoghurt, plain, low-fat	0.23
Mushrooms, raw	0.22
Beans, baked	0.20
Rice, brown, long-grain, boiled	0.15
Broccoli, boiled, drained	0.13
Avocados, raw	0.12
Apricots, raw	0.07
Beetroot (beets) boiled, drained	0.06
Carrots, boiled, drained	0.06
Potatoes, peeled, boiled	0.05
Oranges, raw	0.05
Aubergine (eggplant) boiled, drained	0.04
Bananas, raw	0.04
Onions, boiled, drained	0.04
Peppers, sweet, green, raw	0.04
Cabbage, boiled, drained	0.04
Apples, raw with skin	0.01

Source: USDA National Nutrient Database for Standard Reference, Release 28

L-Arginine

What does the body use arginine for?

- Making tissues, hormones, sperm (in males) and other types of protein
- Helping wounds to heal
- Stimulating the pancreas to release insulin
- Helping to remove excess ammonia
- Stimulating the thymus gland (part of the immune system)
- Making nitric oxide which relaxes blood vessels
- Helps to neutralize the superoxide free radical
- Precursor of creatine, and polyamines.

Arginine is one of the urea cycle amino acids. This means that it plays an important role in turning ammonia into urea, a substance which can be excreted via the kidneys. Ammonia, which is toxic to the brain and to energy production, is formed when proteins are broken down in the body.

Arginine also forms part of antidiuretic hormone, which helps to regulate the kidneys and the blood pressure. Other hormones which depend on arginine include insulin, glucagon and growth hormone.

What foods is it found in?

- Gelatine
- Peanuts
- Almonds, pumpkin seeds, sunflower seeds, Brazil nuts
- Meat, fish
- Oats and other grains

Useful information

Research suggests that arginine supplements are effective in

- Regulating blood pressure[1]
- Improving sports performance[2,3,4]
- Improving blood sugar balance[5,6,7]
- Improving diabetic complications[8,9]
- Increasing the distance which can be walked pain-free by those suffering from artery problems and high cholesterol[10]
- Improving glaucoma—a disease that can cause blindness—by regulating the pressure within the eyes[11]

Arginine's ability to help high blood pressure, angina and other heart problems, and (in men) the erectile dysfunction that can accompany these disorders, is due to its important role in nitric oxide production. (NB: arginine will not help erectile dysfunction caused by blood pressure medication or by psychological factors).

Blood pressure

To investigate the effects of L-arginine-rich diets six healthy volunteers (with an average age of 39 years) received at random, a normal diet (Diet 1), a diet containing arginine-rich foods (Diet 2), or a normal diet plus L-arginine supplements (Diet 3). All had the same sodium intake. After one week, Diets 2 and 3 resulted in blood pressure reductions of 6.2 mm Hg systolic/5 mm Hg diastolic, and 6.2 mm Hg systolic/6.8 mm Hg diastolic respectively. There was also a slight increase in creatinine clearance and in fasting blood glucose. Serum total cholesterol and triglyceride (blood fats) decreased and HDL (good) cholesterol increased after Diet 2, but not after Diet 3. These results indicate that a moderate increase in L-arginine significantly lowers blood pressure and assists kidney function and carbohydrate metabolism in healthy volunteers[1].

Kidneys

Some kidney specialists point out that arginine plays many roles in kidney function, and is of therapeutic value in a number of kidney diseases induced in experimental animals, including enlarged kidneys due to protein over-feeding, and diabetic nephropathy. They suggest that L-arginine supplements could be of value for many human kidney diseases[12].

In one study, an amino acid supplement containing glycine, L-aspartic acid, L-glutamic acid, L-glutamine, L-histidine and L-arginine was administered daily to patients with kidney failure on a low-protein diet. After one year of supplementation, significant improvements in glomerular filtration and creatinine clearance rates were found. The improvements were maintained after the supplementation ceased[13].

Senility

L-arginine supplements at a dose of 1.6 grams/day were administered for three months to 16 elderly nursing home patients with an average age of 79 years. Cognitive function (mental ability) increased in all patients from a score of 16 to 23. Three months after the end of arginine treatment the score returned to 17. While on the treatment, the patients also showed more expressive faces and quicker responses. There were no side effects[14].

Clear airways

The cilia are minute hairs in the walls of the bronchial air passages leading to our lungs, which constantly sweep upwards unwanted debris such as dust and smoke particles so that they can be expelled. In an unusual experiment, 10 patients with genetically defective cilia and 10 normal people were administered three grams of nasally-inhaled arginine dissolved in 10 ml of salt solution by means of a nebulizer. In both groups the activity of the cilia and the rate of mucus clearance was significantly increased. This seems to suggest that arginine can help to protect our lungs and airways by speeding up their cleaning process[15].

Growth hormone and body-building

Growth hormone declines by 10-15% in each decade of advancing age. It is thought that this decline contributes to reduced musculoskeletal mass, increased obesity, and loss of cognitive function in the elderly. L-arginine has been shown to promote growth hormone release[16].

Many people take arginine (plus another amino acid, ornithine) as a body-building supplement, since increased levels of growth hormone may help to increase muscle bulk. Dr Eric Braverman, author of the *Healing Nutrients Within,* suggests that ornithine is a better arginine supplement than arginine itself, because it enters the mitochondria (the energy-producing part of the cell) more readily than arginine. The body readily converts ornithine to arginine. Some research suggests that increases in lean body mass and strength can be achieved with just one gram a day of each amino acid[17].

L-arginine has also been shown to stimulate fat breakdown and the expression of key genes responsible for activating fatty acid oxidation to CO_2 and water. Both animal studies and human studies on patients with type II diabetes show that supplementation with arginine effectively reduces white adipose tissue. There is great interest in this supplement's potential for the prevention and treatment of metabolic syndrome[18].

Sports performance

L-arginine supplementation is being used by athletes to enhance tissue growth and general performance, to increase ergogenic potential, muscle tolerance to high intensity exercise and gas exchange threshold; to decrease ammonia and lessen the recovery period, and to improve wound healing[19].

A supplement combination of branched-chain amino acids and arginine may be able to improve performance in trained athletes by alleviating fatigue following bursts of intense activity[2].

Non-athletes and even individuals with congestive heart failure may also be able to improve their exercise or physical work capacity by taking arginine supplements[3,4].

Insulin sensitivity

Visceral obesity (apple-shape body) is linked with poor insulin sensitivity, also known as insulin resistance, leading to high insulin levels which make it extremely difficult to lose weight. Researchers have found that three months of L-arginine supplementation can improve insulin sensitivity in patients with visceral obesity[5,6]. This is very encouraging as insulin resistance is a precursor to type II diabetes.

After eight weeks of arginine supplements at 6 grams per day to obese individuals, the average reduction in waist circumference was 7 cm (2.75 inches)[7].

According to some research, arginine supplementation can reverse metabolic syndrome—a pre-diabetic condition[20].

Diabetic complications

L-arginine supplementation improves vascular (blood vessel) function in diabetics, and is becoming an important tool for the treatment of diabetic complications, including diabetic kidney disease[8,9].

Because of its involvement in numerous areas of human biochemistry, arginine in supplement form has also been used in therapeutic regimes for angina pectoris, congestive heart failure, chronic kidney disease, coronary heart disease, pregnancy preeclampsia, and erectile dysfunction. It has also been studied in the treatment of HIV/AIDS, burns and trauma, cancer, diabetes and syndrome X, gastrointestinal diseases, male and female infertility, interstitial cystitis, lowered immunity, and senile dementia[21,22,23].

SUPPLEMENTS

How to use arginine supplements

Body-building

1-2 grams taken 2-3 times a day on an empty stomach, five days a week in combination with weight training.

Supporting nitric oxide production

1,500 mg of arginine per day for at least six months, plus a handful of nuts or seeds daily.

How safe are arginine supplements?

In trials which administer arginine supplementation, single doses of 3-6 grams rarely provoke side effects. Gastroinestinal symptoms have been reported at doses of more than 9 grams, with healthy athletes appearing to be more susceptible than diabetic patients[24].

While one study suggests that arginine supplementation should be avoided by individuals with breast cancer,[25] another suggests that arginine supplements may may have a role in the treatment of breast cancer.[26]

High levels of arginine (from food or supplements) are thought to encourage the growth of viruses belonging to the herpes family, so people who suffer from shingles or recurrent herpes virus sores may find that this problem is aggravated when they eat a lot of arginine-rich foods. People suffering from chronic fatigue syndrome may be infected with the Epstein-Barr virus, which is a member of the herpes virus family. These people too may benefit from caution with arginine consumption. See also L-Lysine.

Arginine content of common foods in grams per 100g

Food	Arginine (g)
Gelatine, dry	6.62
Pumpkin and squash seed kernels, roasted	5.28
Peanuts, dry roasted	2.83
Almonds, raw	2.47
Sunflower seeds, hulled	2.40
Brazil nuts, raw	2.39
Walnuts, raw	2.28
Prawns, boiled	1.83
Tuna, skipjack, fresh, raw	1.32
Chicken meat, raw	1.29
Pork, composite of various cuts, trimmed, raw	1.20
Oats	1.19
Salmon, Atlantic, farmed, raw	1.19
Beef, ground, extra-lean (approx. 21% fat)	1.19
Herring, Atlantic, raw	1.08
Cheese, cheddar	0.94
Buckwheat flour, whole groat	0.94
Chick peas, boiled	0.84
Eggs, hard-boiled	0.76
Lentils, boiled	0.70
Wheat flour, whole-grain	0.64
Tofu, raw, with calcium sulphate	0.54
Cornmeal, whole-grain, yellow	0.41
Beans, baked	0.30
Rice, brown, long-grain, boiled	0.20
Onions, boiled, drained	0.18
Yoghurt, plain, low-fat	0.16
Broccoli, boiled, drained	0.16
Mushrooms, raw	0.14
Potatoes, peeled, boiled	0.08
Oranges, raw	0.07
Avocados, raw	0.06
Cabbage, boiled, drained	0.06
Bananas, raw	0.05
Aubergine (eggplant) boiled, drained	0.05
Carrots, boiled, drained	0.05
Beetroot (beets) boiled, drained	0.04
Peppers, sweet, green, raw	0.04
Apples, raw with skin	0.01

Source: USDA National Nutrient Database for Standard Reference, Release 28

Aspartates (aspartic acid)

What does the body use aspartic acid for?

- Helping to remove excess ammonia
- DNA metabolism
- Energy production
- Excitatory neurotransmitter
- Stimulating thymus gland, bone marrow and spleen
- Energy production
- With glutamine, aspartic acid forms asparagine, needed to stimulate the secretion of glucagon
- With citrulline, aspartic acid forms arginosuccinate, needed to break ammonia down to urea.

Aspartic acid plays an important role in converting ammonia into urea, which can be excreted via the kidneys. Ammonia is a brain toxin produced by protein breakdown.

Aspartic acid is also a major excitatory neurotransmitter, which means that it helps electrical impulses to pass along nerves, to muscles, organs etc.

Research shows that both potassium and magnesium aspartates support the tissues of the thymus gland, bone marrow and spleen, and help the red blood cell-producing organs to regenerate after exposure to radiation.

If necessary, aspartic acid can be turned into glucose, thus acting as a source of energy for the body. It also plays a role in oxidative phosphorylation, one of the steps in energy production.

What foods is it found in?

- Gelatine
- Peanuts
- Almonds, sunflower seeds
- Meat, fish
- Walnuts

Aspartic acid is also made within the body from another amino acid, glutamic acid, by means of enzymes which use vitamin B6.

Sports endurance

A number of researchers have carried out studies (mostly on animals) to find out whether aspartate supplementation can improve exercise capacity, There is some evidence of a glycogen-sparing action, and reduced lactic acid and ammonia, but studies have shown conflicting results. Aspartate has not been shown to increase muscle endurance or strength[1].

SUPPLEMENTS

Aspartic acid is not sold in its pure form. It can be taken as mineral aspartates, such as magnesium aspartate.

Aspartic acid content of common foods in grams per 100g

Gelatine, dry	5.27
Peanuts, dry roasted	2.89
Almonds, raw	2.73
Sunflower seeds, hulled	2.45
Tuna, skipjack, fresh, raw	2.25
Prawns, boiled	2.16
Salmon, Atlantic, farmed, raw	2.04
Chicken meat, raw	1.91
Herring, Atlantic, raw	1.84
Walnuts, raw	1.83
Pork, composite of various cuts, trimmed, raw	1.74
Beef, ground, extra-lean (approx. 21% fat)	1.62
Cheese, cheddar	1.60
Oats	1.45
Brazil nuts, raw	1.36
Eggs, hard-boiled	1.26
Buckwheat flour, whole groat	1.08
Chick peas, boiled	1.04
Lentils, boiled	1.00
Tofu, raw, with calcium sulphate	0.89
Wheat flour, whole-grain	0.70
Beans, baked	0.58
Cornmeal, whole-grain, yellow	0.57
Potatoes, peeled, boiled	0.42
Yoghurt, plain, low-fat	0.42
Apricots, raw	0.31
Avocados, raw	0.28
Mushrooms, raw	0.27
Rice, brown, long-grain, boiled	0.24
Broccoli, boiled, drained	0.23
Carrots, boiled, drained	0.14
Aubergine (eggplant) boiled, drained	0.13
Peppers, sweet, green, raw	0.13
Beetroot (beets) boiled, drained	0.12
Oranges, raw	0.11
Bananas, raw	0.11
Cabbage, boiled, drained	0.10
Onions, boiled, drained	0.07
Apples, raw with skin	0.03

Source: USDA National Nutrient Database for Standard Reference, Release 28

Carnitine and Acetyl L-carnitine (ALC)

What does the body use carnitine for?

- Releasing energy from fat
- Production of body heat
- Turning amino acids into fuel for energy
- Controlling ketone levels in the blood
- Elimination of xenobiotic substances (chemicals and toxins)[1]

The most important function of carnitine is thought to be its role in helping to make fat into energy by carrying fat across the outer membrane to the energy-making parts (the mitochondria) of each cell. The more carnitine is available, the faster fat is transported, and the more fat is used for energy. The muscles and heart especially benefit from this source of energy. The heart contains more carnitine than any other organ of the body. 'Brown' fat, a type of body fat which contains a lot of mitochondria and is responsible for the production of much body heat, is especially dependent on carnitine.

Carnitine also ensures regeneration of coenzyme A, a key element in energy production.

Carnitine helps the body to break down branched-chain amino acids into fuel for the muscles when needed, and it controls ketone levels in the blood. Ketones are formed when fats used for energy production are not completely oxidized. They are high in diabetics, and give rise to the acetone odour noticed in the breath of those in a diabetic coma. Ketone levels also rise with high-protein or high-fat diets and during weight loss regimes. They tend to acidify the blood.

Acetyl L-carnitine (ALC) is a form of carnitine which is thought to be better assimilated into the brain. For research into carnitine and heart disease, some research studies have used another form of carnitine known as propionyl carnitine.

What foods is carnitine found in?

- Red meat and liver
- Dairy products
- Yeast

A normal omnivorous diet provides about 50 mg per day of carnitine. Most people do not need to eat much food containing carnitine, since the body makes about 20 mg per day from the amino acids lysine and methionine, with the aid of vitamin B6, vitamin C and iron. However some vegans (strict vegetarians) may consume less than 5 mg of carnitine per day, and rely almost totally on carnitine synthesis for their needs. They should be particularly vigilant that their diet provides enough carnitine precursors[2]. Lysine and methionine are not abundant in most plant foods.

Useful information

Carnitine deficiency is common[1]. It can occur

- If the enzymes which make it are not working efficiently or are not properly supplied with all necessary materials,

- If there is an excessive demand on carnitine due to high ketone or ammonia levels
- In severe liver disease.

Fatigue

It is now well established that carnitine supplements can make muscles more efficient when exercising, and can reduce the amount of lactic acid produced by exercising. (Lactic acid is responsible for muscle ache after exercise.) Lactic acid levels are also high in sufferers of chronic fatigue syndrome, also known as M.E. In a study on 30 chronic fatigue patients, there were improvements in 12 out of the 18 symptoms and parameters measured after eight weeks of treatment with carnitine. The greatest improvement took place between four and eight weeks of treatment. Only one patient was unable to complete the full course of treatment due to diarrhoea[3].

The heart

The heart muscle uses fat as its primary energy source. Carnitine is needed to release energy from fat, so it is an absolutely essential nutrient for normal heart function. With ageing, the decline of carnitine plays a role in the weakening of the heart's muscles.

People who have suffered heart attacks or people with congestive heart failure have especially low carnitine levels and are at risk of repeat heart attacks or early death. In a study on patients who had suffered a heart attack, those supplementing with carnitine had a death rate of just 1.2% in the year, while 12.5% of control patients (those not taking the supplement) died, with the majority of deaths attributed to repeat heart attacks[4].

Carnitine supplements have also been used to:

- Reduce angina by improving the circulation through the heart[5]
- Increase the pain-free walking distance in intermittent claudication (a painful condition of the legs, which is linked with heart and artery disease)[6]
- Reduce the risk of developing congestive heart failure after a heart attack[7]
- Improve the symptoms and extend the life of people with congestive heart failure[8]

Diabetics and kidney patients on dialysis are at especially high risk for cardiovascular complications and early death and may benefit from carnitine supplements.

Alzheimer's disease

Acetyl L-carnitine (ALC) can enhance the production of acetylcholine, an important neurotransmitter needed for memory. It can also help to clear the waste products of energy metabolism. Research has shown that ALC supplementation at the rate of about two grams a day can help to slow down the progress of Alzheimer's disease and reverse mental decline[9,10].

Most forms of age-related memory and cognitive decline are closely related to dysfunction in the mitochondria in brain tissue. Carnitine plays an important role in mitochondrial function. Studies have shown that geriatric patients supplemented with 1.5 to 2 grams of acetyl-L-carnitine daily show marked improvements in mental status and memory scores[11].

Weight loss

One of the most popular uses of carnitine supplements is as a weight loss aid.

In one study, 18 overweight adolescents were given nutrition education, a physical training programme and a calorie-controlled diet, and some were also given 2 grams of L-carnitine per day for three months. Those on carnitine lost on average 4.6 kg more than the rest, and the most overweight ones had a 25 per cent greater weight loss. In another study, administering only 200 mg of L-carnitine per day, there was still a significant loss of body fat, as well as a reduction in total cholesterol and LDL ('bad') cholesterol. The subjects had more energy, were less hungry, and had less cravings for sugar. Carnitine aids weight loss by increase the ability to use fat for energy[12]. Some researchers have found that those taking carnitine supplements are able to burn fat 22% faster than control patients[13].

Physical performance

L-carnitine supplements are popular with athletes, although conflicting results have been found in research into their ability to enhance endurance performance. Recent studies have shown that L-carnitine supplementation can decrease free radical generation, muscle soreness and hypoxic stress-related tissue damage caused by exercise, and aid the recovery process[14,15].

Fertility

Supplementation with L-carnitine and/or acetyl-L-carnitine can improve sperm count, motility, straight-swimming ability, and total normal sperm forms. In research investigating the effects of carnitine supplementation on male fertility, fertility-challenged couples experienced pregnancy rates of 21.8 per cent in the carnitine group but only 1.7 per cent in the control group[16].

Thyroid

In the condition known as hyperthyroidism, where abnormally high levels of thyroid hormone cause symptoms such as rapid heart beat, bone thinning, sleeplessness and palpitations, it has also been observed that carnitine levels in the muscles are reduced, and patients experience muscle weakness. Some researchers have found that these problems can be mitigated by administering 2-4 grams a day of carnitine supplements. These supplements are not a cure for the condition, but can help to reduce some of its harmful consequences[17].

Hearing

By reducing mutations in mitochondrial DNA, acetyl-L-carnitine supplementation has been found to help prevent noise-induced hearing loss and also age-related hearing loss. Much like n-acetyl cysteine, acetyl-L-carnitine appears to be effective even when administered after exposure to loud noise[18,19].

SUPPLEMENTS

How to use carnitine supplements

Carnitine is an expensive supplement. A dosage of 500 mg per day would provide a similar amount of carnitine to a small portion of red meat. This can be safely taken if you are not sure whether your body is making enough carnitine for your needs. You can also experiment with up to 2,000 mg a day and then cut back to the minimum dose which seems to work well for you. Try acetyl-L-carnitine (ALC) supplements (500-1000 mg per day) instead if your priority is to support your brainpower and memory.

Supplementation with choline significantly reduces the excretion of carnitine in the urine and so can help to keep up carnitine levels in the body. Choline supplements (best taken in the form of lecithin) are considerably cheaper than carnitine and may help a low dose of carnitine to achieve the same effects as a high one[20].

How safe are carnitine supplements?

In the above-mentioned studies, the researchers concluded that L-carnitine supplements are safe and very well tolerated[3]. ALC product labels usually indicate that this form of carnitine should be avoided by pregnant or breastfeeding women. Excessive doses of L-carnitine supplements may cause digestive discomfort and occasionally a body odour.

Carnitine content of common foods per 100g

Lamb	190 mg
Beef steak	95 mg
Ground beef	94 mg
Pork	27.7 mg
Bacon	23.3 mg
Tempeh	19.5 mg
Cod fish	5.6 mg
Chicken breast	3.9 mg
American cheese	3.7 mg
Ice cream	3.7 mg
Whole milk	3.3 mg
Avocado (one whole)	2.0mg
Cottage cheese	1.1 mg
Whole-wheat bread	0.36 mg
Asparagus	0.19 mg
White bread	0.14 mg
Macaroni	0.12 mg
Peanut butter	0.08mg
Rice (cooked)	0.04 mg
Egg	0.01 mg
Orange juice	0.00 mg
Lentil	2.1 mg
Potato	2.4 mg
Sweet Potato	1.1 mg
Banana	0.2 mg
Carrot	0.3 mg
Apple (without skin)	0.2 mg
Raisin	0.8 mg

Source: Demarquoy J et al, Radioisotopic determination of L-carnitine content in foods commonly eaten in Western countries. Food Chemistry 86 (1): 137–142.

L-Cysteine and n-acetyl cysteine

What does the body use cysteine for?

- Making taurine and glutathione
- Providing special links that hold proteins together
- Cysteine can be turned into glucose if necessary
- Helps to synthesize fatty acids
- With methionine, helps to make lipoic acid
- Helps to make fingernails, hair and outer skin layers (once transformed into cystine)
- Has antioxidant properties
- Binds to heavy metals such as mercury and hastens their removal.

Cysteine belongs to the sulphur group of amino acids. For most purposes it can be considered the same as cystine, an amino acid formed by two molecules of cysteine combining together. (Cystine helps to give structure to proteins.)

Together with pantothenic acid (vitamin B5) cysteine helps to form coenzyme A, a key element in energy production.

In the liver, blood plasma and bronchial tubes of the lungs, n-acetyl cysteine (NAC) creates reduced glutathione—the most active form of the amino acid glutathione which neutralizes harmful free radicals. Cysteine is also needed to make the detoxifying amino acid taurine.

What foods is cysteine found in?

- Sunflower seeds
- Oats
- Brazil nuts
- Wheatgerm
- Soy flour
- Peanuts
- Eggs

Cysteine can also be synthesized from methionine.

Detoxification

A cysteine or methionine deficiency can result in allergy-like symptoms caused by sensitivities to chemicals. These sensitivities stem from sluggish liver function—a reduced ability to convert the chemicals into harmless substances which can be excreted. Practitioners of environmental medicine specialize in helping people with these problems by correcting their deficiencies of cysteine, glutathione and other important liver nutrients. Given by mouth or intravenously, NAC is the standard treatment for paracetamol (acetaminophen) overdose and helps the liver to break down a variety of other toxic compounds, including carbon tetrachloride, acrylonitriles, halothane, paraquat, acetaldehyde, and residues of drugs after cancer chemotherapy. It is also especially useful for helping to remove excess copper, lead, mercury or arsenic from the body.

Cysteine levels are usually abnormally low in people diagnosed as HIV-positive. This suggests that there are abnormally high demands on cysteine here—probably by the liver—and researchers have obtained beneficial results from supplementing these people with NAC and other key nutrients needed for liver support[1].

Diabetes and insulin resistance

Diabetics too may benefit from cysteine since it is required to make lipoic acid, a substance which can help to prevent complications in diabetes, and can reduce the need for insulin. Cysteine is also needed to make special links that hold the insulin molecule together.

Insulin resistance is a condition where insulin does not work properly, so the body keeps making more and more of it, leading to high insulin levels that throw the body's hormones out of balance. It is a pre-diabetic condition, and blood sugar levels may also be raised. One of the proposed causes of insulin resistance in obese individuals is glycation—a reaction between the body's proteins and high levels of blood sugar. Glycation products are also consumed in food when meat is browned at high temperatures. Glycation and its products (known as AGEs) cause much damage to the body's proteins, and in diabetics can lead to complications such as damage to the nerves, eyes, kidneys and heart. Glycation products cause the formation of free radicals, which inhibit the uptake of glucose by cells. Researchers believe that glycation is involved in the development of obesity-related insulin resistance. In one study the effects of AGEs on glucose uptake were completely reversed by treatment with n-acetyl cysteine[2].

Respiratory problems and COPD

NAC has the unusual property of being able to dissolve thick mucus and may also act as an expectorant by stimulating the cilia (minute hairs which continually sweep our airways) and lung reflexes, so clearing the mucus from the airways. It has been used in research studies to treat chronic obstructive pulmonary disease (COPD) and bronchitis[3].

Researchers believe that the benefits of NAC supplementation against COPD lie in its antioxidant properties. Oxidative stress caused by airway inflammation is increased in COPD and may account for the progressive deterioration of structure and function of the respiratory tract observed in this disease. NAC supplementation at a dose of 600 mg administered twice a day for 2 months rapidly reduces the oxidative stress burden in the airways of stable COPD patients[4].

NAC treatment can also have benefits against air trapping in COPD patients, and improve their physical performance[5].

Influenza

One interesting use of NAC supplementation is against influenza. In one study, NAC supplements were shown to inhibit flu virus replication and virus-induced inflammation[6].

Cancers

NAC is currently one of the most intensely researched anti-cancer substances. Test tube studies have shown NAC to be able to block the harmful effects of many cancer-causing agents and to inhibit the growth of some types of cancer cells, including melanoma and prostate cancer[7]. In both test tube and animal studies, NAC selectively protects normal cells, but not malignant ones, from chemotherapy and radiation toxicity. This effect is due to its antioxidant functions—its ability to neutralize free radicals produced during treatment. These free radicals are responsible for many of the side effects experienced. Often, antioxidant therapy does not interfere with chemotherapy because the chemotherapy drugs do not depend on free radicals for their effectiveness. But cysteine and other antioxidants can still interfere with the action of some chemotherapy drugs, and expertise is required in selecting the right antioxidants[8].

Ear problems and hearing

In one study, NAC was instilled into the ears of children after treatment for otitis media (accumulation of fluid in the middle ear). This significantly reduced the number of episodes of ear problems and lengthened the time between recurrences of the otitis media[9].

NAC supplements have also been used to reduce hearing damage in those exposed to military or industrial noise[10,11].

Duodenal ulcers

The use of DL-cysteine in preventing the recurrence of duodenal ulcers was compared with placebo (an inert substance) and with cimetidine, the conventional anti-ulcer medication. After one year the relapse rate was 64 per cent for placebo patients, 30 per cent for cimetidine patients, and only 11 per cent for cysteine patients[12].

Polycystic ovaries

Polycystic ovary syndrome (PCOS) is strongly associated with insulin resistance. NAC supplementation has been found very helpful to improve insulin sensitivity in patients with this condition[13].

A combined supplement of NAC and L-arginine may even be able to restore menstrual function and ovulation in PCOS. This effect is attributed to an improvement in insulin sensitivity[14].

Because of the insulin resistance factor, many physicians are treating PCOS with the diabetes drug metformin. In a study comparing NAC supplements with metformin, NAC was found to be equally effective in reducing symptoms of PCOS[15].

Bipolar disorder

In a study on bipolar disorder, patients were given 1 gram of NAC twice a day. After eight weeks, effectiveness scores were medium to high for nine out of twelve criteria measured[16]. It is thought that these improvements may have occurred because cysteine raises glutathione levels, which are usually low in bipolar disorder.

SUPPLEMENTS

How to use cysteine supplements

For most purposes the suggested dose is 500 mg three times a day, which is equivalent to the amount of cysteine in 400 grams of porridge oats. According to Eric Braverman author of the excellent amino acid bible, the *Healing Nutrients Within,* L-cysteine supplements are probably just as good for most purposes as the more expensive NAC supplements although most of the medical research has been carried out with NAC. Supplements need to be taken three times a day because peak plasma levels occur approximately one hour after an oral dose and 12 hours after the dose they are undetectable in the blood plasma. Cysteine and lysine fight each other for absorption so are best not taken at the same time.

Another form of cysteine supplement is based on whey protein concentrate. This has been used in medical studies to raise glutathione levels by up to 35 per cent in white blood cells[17] and has also been found to reduce muscle fatigue and boost muscular performance in sports medicine[18]. There are also many reports that it has an anti-tumour effect against cancers of the prostate, uterus, kidney and bladder at a dose of 10-30 grams daily[19].

How safe are cysteine supplements?

Cysteine and methionine are converted to homocysteine, a toxic amino acid which has been linked with heart and artery disease and osteoporosis. In most people homocysteine is quickly broken down and rendered harmless by two enzymes, but a few individuals require extra large amounts of B vitamins to support these enzymes when extra cysteine or methionine are consumed. If you need to supplement with these amino acids, it is wise to take B vitamin supplements at the same time, especially folic acid and vitamins B6 and B12.

NAC supplements prescribed in large amounts as a paracetamol (acetaminophen) antidote have increased the excretion of copper and zinc, so these minerals should be supplemented if taking NAC on a long-term basis. NAC can also interact with some pharmaceutical medications. No side effects have been reported by researchers, except in one study, where the participants reported reactions such as dry mouth and vomiting. Since participants in other studies have not reported such effects, they may have been due to ingredients other than NAC in the product.

Chronic fatigue researcher Dr Paul Cheney does not recommend NAC supplements for people with a severe glutathione deficiency, which is common in chronic fatigue syndrome.

Cysteine supplementation may worsen symptoms of intestinal candidiasis, because Candida can metabolize cysteine easily.

Cysteine, glutathione and lipoic acid supplements must never be administered at the same time as radiotherapy for cancer, since they are such efficient antioxidants that they would interfere with its effectiveness. They may also be able to interfere with the action of certain chemotherapy agents.

In the table opposite, cystine figures are given because cysteine figures are not available.

Cystine content of common foods in grams per 100 g

Wheatgerm, raw	0.46
Sunflower seeds, hulled	0.45
Oats	0.41
Brazil nuts, raw	0.35
Wheat flour, whole-grain	0.32
Peanuts, dry roasted	0.30
Eggs, hard-boiled	0.29
Almonds, raw	0.28
Chicken meat, raw	0.27
Pork, composite of various cuts, trimmed, raw	0.24
Tuna, skipjack, fresh, raw	0.24
Prawns, boiled	0.23
Buckwheat flour, whole groat	0.22
Salmon, Atlantic, farmed, raw	0.21
Walnuts, raw	0.21
Herring, Atlantic, raw	0.19
Beef, ground, extra-lean (approx. 21% fat)	0.17
Cornmeal, whole-grain, yellow	0.15
Cheese, cheddar	0.13
Chick peas, boiled	0.12
Lentils, boiled	0.12
Tofu, raw, with calcium sulphate	0.11
Beans, baked	0.05
Yoghurt, plain, low-fat	0.05
Rice, brown, long-grain, boiled	0.03
Onions, boiled, drained	0.02
Potatoes, peeled, boiled	0.02
Avocados, raw	0.02
Broccoli, boiled, drained	0.02
Beetroot (beets) boiled, drained	0.02
Bananas, raw	0.02
Peppers, sweet, green, raw	0.02
Oranges, raw	0.01
Carrots, boiled, drained	0.01
Mushrooms, raw	0.01
Aubergine (eggplant) boiled, drained	0.00
Apricots, raw	0.00
Apples, raw with skin	0.00
Gelatine, dry	0.00

Source: USDA National Nutrient Database for Standard Reference, Release 28

Gamma-amino butyric acid (GABA)

What does the body use GABA for?

Although not strictly speaking an amino acid, GABA is often classified with the amino acids. It functions as the most widely distributed inhibitory neurotransmitter in the brain, helping to control the passage of electrical impulses along the nerve cells to muscles, organs etc.

What foods is it found in?

GABA is not found in food, but is made from the amino acid glutamic acid.

Useful information

Vitamin B6 and taurine are needed to make GABA, and a B6 deficiency could lead to a GABA deficiency. This could be a factor in epilepsy since GABA is almost always deficient in people who suffer from seizures.

GABA is involved in blood pressure control, so substances which stimulate receptors which respond to GABA are considered useful in combating high blood pressure.

Benzodiazepine tranquillizer drugs (such as Valium), produce their anti-anxiety and muscle-relaxant effects by activating the nerve cells and receptors which respond to GABA. Alcohol consumption leads to increased GABA levels in the brain.

Theanine, an amino acid found in green tea, increases the production of GABA and dopamine and protects the cells of the hippocampus—the seat of learning and memory in the brain—from damage[1]. Theanine easily crosses the blood-brain barrier and produces a calming effect on the brain.

Sleep

The herb lemon balm contains an ingredient that slows the natural breakdown of GABA in the body and promotes a deeper, better sleep[2].

Hops are considered a sedative and have been found to increase GABA activity[3].

Tapering off psychiatric medications

GABA can help with mood instability if supplemented while tapering off psychiatric medications (with your doctor's permission, of course). Taking it several hours before bedtime can also help with sleep. GABA is said to be especially useful for patients tapering from lithium.

There are some case reports that individuals with severe anxiety can stop using diazepam and replace lorazepam with 200 mg of GABA four times each day[4].

SUPPLEMENTS

How to use GABA supplements

The following conditions may be linked with a GABA deficiency. If other methods have not proved helpful, GABA supplements may be able to combat them:

- Anxiety and panic attacks
- Epilepsy and seizures

Dosage: 500-1000 mg per day, taken on an empty stomach. (Some practitioners recommend up to 2 to 3 grams daily.) Since GABA supplements are expensive, it is useful to know that supplementation with the amino acid taurine increases the body's breakdown of glutamate to GABA.

How safe are GABA supplements?

Product labels should indicate that GABA supplements should not be taken at the same time as tranquillizers. Excessive supplementation with GABA may occasionally lead to temporary symptoms of increased heart rate or shortness of breath.

Glutamic acid (glutamate)

What does the body use glutamic acid for?

- Neurotransmitter
- Transporting ammonia to the liver for processing
- Making other amino acids
- Making folate (folic acid) - an important B vitamin

Glutamic acid is the most common excitatory neurotransmitter, (assisting electrical impulses to travel along nerves) and is found in particularly high levels in the prostate gland and in the memory centre and other parts of the brain. It is also used to make other amino acids, including proline, ornithine, arginine, glutamine, glutathione and GABA. Glutamine is formed when glutamic acid combines with ammonia.

What foods is it found in?

- Gelatine
- Cheese
- Sunflower seeds
- Almonds, peanuts
- Wheat flour

43 per cent of wheat gluten consists of glutamic acid, and 23 per cent of milk protein. Glutamic acid or glutamate can also be manufactured by the body.

Useful information

Researchers working with epileptic patients have found that most epileptics have decreased taurine, GABA and glycine, but increased aspartic acid and glutamic acid. This imbalance may be due to a vitamin B6 deficiency. The enzyme glutamate decarboxylase, without which glutamic acid cannot be broken down into GABA, requires adequate levels of vitamin B6. Since both epileptics and people with severe vitamin B6 deficiency suffer from convulsions, some people with B6 deficiency may be mistakenly diagnosed as epileptics.

'Chinese restaurant syndrome', the symptoms of which include headache, nausea, weakness, flushing and sweating after eating Chinese food, may be due to a high content of monosodium glutamate—a sodium salt of glutamic acid—in the food. It has been proposed that this syndrome is caused by abnormally high vitamin B6 needs in certain individuals, and can be prevented with vitamin B6 supplementation since B6 supports the enzyme which breaks down glutamate. High levels of glutamate in the body are undesirable because they lead to destruction of glutathione and triggering of cell death.

SUPPLEMENTS

Since large amounts of glutamic acid are found in food, supplements are not normally on sale.

Glutamic acid content of common foods in grams/100g

Gelatine, dry	8.75
Cheese, cheddar	6.09
Sunflower seeds, hulled	5.58
Almonds, raw	5.17
Peanuts, dry roasted	4.95
Wheat flour, whole-grain	4.33
Oats	3.71
Prawns, boiled	3.57
Tuna, skipjack, fresh, raw	3.28
Chicken meat, raw	3.20
Brazil nuts, raw	3.15
Salmon, Atlantic, farmed, raw	2.97
Pork, composite of various cuts, trimmed, raw	2.92
Walnuts, raw	2.82
Beef, ground, extra-lean (approx. 21% fat)	2.78
Herring, Atlantic, raw	2.68
Buckwheat flour, whole groat	1.95
Eggs, hard-boiled	1.64
Chick peas, boiled	1.55
Cornmeal, whole-grain, yellow	1.53
Lentils, boiled	1.40
Tofu, raw, with calcium sulphate	1.40
Yoghurt, plain, low-fat	1.03
Beans, baked	0.73
Rice, brown, long-grain, boiled	0.53
Mushrooms, raw	0.50
Beetroot (beets) boiled, drained	0.45
Broccoli, boiled, drained	0.40
Potatoes, peeled, boiled	0.29
Cabbage, boiled, drained	0.22
Onions, boiled, drained	0.22
Carrots, boiled, drained	0.21
Avocados, raw	0.21
Apricots, raw	0.16
Aubergine (eggplant) boiled, drained	0.15
Peppers, sweet, green, raw	0.12
Bananas, raw	0.11
Oranges, raw	0.09
Apples, raw with skin	0.02

Source: USDA National Nutrient Database for Standard Reference, Release 28

L-Glutamine

What does the body use glutamine for?

- Involved in more metabolic processes than any other amino acid
- Can be turned into glucose if necessary
- Source of energy for the brain
- Source of energy for cells lining the intestines
- Helps to make GABA, glutamate and glutathione
- Helps to make vitamin B3 (niacin)
- Helps in DNA synthesis
- Helps to break down uric acid
- Acts as an ammonia carrier in the nervous system

Glutamine is glutamic acid combined with free ammonia nitrogen, and is the major vehicle for nitrogen transfer among tissues. It protects the body (especially the nervous system) from high levels of ammonia by accepting and then releasing ammonia to form other amino acids and nitrogen-containing substances. This is important since excess ammonia plays a major part in the development of degenerative diseases of the nervous system by interfering with the metabolism of neurons (nerve cells).

Glutamine makes up 60% of the amino acids in the body and is the most abundant amino acid in the blood, where its concentration is three to four times greater than all other amino acids. In fasting or starvation states, when stored carbohydrate (glycogen) has been exhausted, large amounts of glutamine and alanine are released from the muscles and serve to shuttle nitrogen and carbon (derived from amino acids) to other tissues. The carbon can be converted to glucose by the liver and used to produce energy.

The brain can use glutamine instead of glucose as a source of energy. Glutamine is particularly abundant in the cerebrospinal fluid and in the parts of the brain known as the substantia nigra and thalamus. The substantia nigra releases dopamine, and the thalamus, which is controlled by dopamine, is involved in the control of body movements, and also plays a part in sensations and in linking sensations to emotions. Parkinson's disease results from degeneration of the substantia nigra and its ability to release dopamine.

Glutamine plays an important role in maintaining the integrity of the intestinal cells and has been used to prevent and treat a 'leaky gut', which is one of the prime causes of food intolerances[1].

What foods is glutamine found in?

Very little reliable information can be found. Glutamine figures are not given in standard reference works, and some authors claim that glutamine is not found in food. However, one authority says that glutamine is found in quite large amounts in potatoes[2]. The richest food source of glutamine is said to be germinated barley foodstuff, which is made from brewer's spent grain. Cabbage is also rich in glutamine. Other good sources include poultry, beef, fish, beets and dairy products.

Glutamine is primarily made within the body from glutamic acid, arginine, ornithine and proline.

Alcoholism

In the 1960s an experiment was carried out supplementing 15 grams a day of L-glutamine to alcoholics[3]. Compared with a placebo (dummy substance), this seemed to control alcohol consumption quite significantly, but it was many years before research was carried out to investigate these findings further.

It is now known that people going through alcohol withdrawal have decreased dopamine function, and decreased endorphins, which may be a major cause of withdrawal symptoms and relapses. To investigate whether amino acid supplementation could correct these deficits, 20 people suffering from alcohol addiction and beginning a detox programme were given supplements of D-phenylalanine, L-glutamine and 5-hydroxytryptophan (5-HTP) in a 2011 study. D-phenylalanine slows the action of enzymes which break down endorphins, while L-glutamine and 5-HTP help to replenish dopamine. This therapy resulted in a significant decrease in psychiatric symptom scores and alleviation of withdrawal symptoms compared with the control group (the group receiving no treatment)[4].

Critical illness and weight loss

Glutamine is a major 'food' for immune cells and may be the chief reason that muscle tissue decreases during illness, since glutamine is made and stored in muscle. During illness, concentrations can be rapidly depleted as glutamine is sequestered for use in organ and immune function. Key immune cells show a sharp decline in function as glutamine levels are depleted. In the seriously ill, blood glutamine levels are inversely related to health outcomes.

Studies with glutamine-enriched nutrition show beneficial effects on nitrogen balance, muscle protein metabolism, intestinal mucosa, and immunity. With adequate glutamine, white blood cells can become up to 26 per cent more efficient at killing bacteria[5]. Glutamine supplementation heals flattened villi (these comprise the absorptive surface of the small intestine) and stimulates the growth of cells lining the intestine[6]. It may also help to reduce the damage to the intestinal lining caused by irritants or toxins[6].

In certain patient categories the addition of glutamine reduces the number of infectious complications, improves long-term survival, and shortens hospital stay, e.g. bone marrow transplantation patients, new-born infants with severely subnormal weight, patients with multiple organ failure, multi-trauma patients[2].

One study found that patients who had major surgery and were given glutamine did not lose muscle mass during the recuperative period, even though they were inactive[7].

So there may be much truth to the 'old wives' tale' that feeding chicken soup to the sick can help them recover, especially in poor communities, where protein may be in short supply. In the words of Tevye in the famous musical *Fiddler on the Roof*: 'As the good book says, when a poor man eats a chicken, one of them is sick'.

Low-calorie diets used for weight loss are well known to cause muscle loss as well as fat loss because the body breaks down both muscle and fat to obtain its energy supplies. Making sure we consume enough glutamine can help to minimize this problem.

Cancer treatment

In a research study where patients on the toxic anti-tumour drug methotrexate were concurrently given large doses of supplementary glutamine, no patient showed any sign of methotrexate toxicity. Except for one, all patients responded to the methotrexate. The researchers concluded that the glutamine supplement helped to ensure that the methotrexate was preferentially taken up by tumour cells rather than normal cells and so may have helped to make it more effective[8].

Despite theories that glutamine may be able to fuel cancer growth, there are several clinical studies which suggest that glutamine supplementation in cancer patients brings clinical improvements without increasing tumour growth[9]. Some report that supplemental glutamine slows tumour growth by enhancing the immune system. Glutamine supplementation also increases natural killer cell activity and anti-inflammatory activity, and helps protect against oxidative stress[10].

Sports

Endurance athletes have decreased plasma glutamine concentrations after prolonged, strenuous exercise. Prolonged exhaustive exercise is known to deplete the immune system and increase susceptibility to infections. Supplementation with glutamine after intensive exercise has been found to decrease the rate of infections[11,12].

Glutamine is sometimes used in body-building, since supplementation may be able to boost growth hormone levels[13].

SUPPLEMENTS

How to use L-glutamine supplements

Glutamine decays rapidly, and it is important to use a brand with a reputation for good quality. 500 mg to 5 grams per day can be taken experimentally to

- Combat alcohol cravings
- Enhance brain alertness
- As a sports aid

How safe are L-glutamine supplements?

A case of mania has been reported in an individual who took 4 grams of L-glutamine per day.

Based on available published human clinical trial data, researchers believe that L-glutamine is safe at intakes up to 14 grams per day[14].

Glutathione

What does the body use glutathione for?

- One of the most important aids to the liver's detoxification work, especially in neutralizing organochlorine pesticides and related substances
- Makes glutathione peroxidase, an enzyme which deactivates harmful peroxides
- Helps to break down excessive insulin in the liver and kidneys
- Helps transport amino acids into and out of cells
- Regulates genes involved in chronic inflammation
- Helps to control levels of hormones and prostaglandins
- Recycles vitamin C within the body

According to Lester Packer PhD, one of the world's foremost antioxidant researchers, maintaining a high level of glutathione is critical for life. The liver and lungs both contain extremely high levels of glutathione. Exposure to toxic chemicals stimulates the secretion of glutathione from the liver into the blood plasma. Once in the plasma, glutathione combines with the toxins. The resultant combination is then converted to mercapturic acid, which can be excreted by the kidneys. Glutathione peroxidase, an enzyme made with glutathione, deactivates hydrogen peroxide, a harmful precursor to free radicals.

Glutathione's role in breaking down excessive insulin is important since excessively high insulin levels will lead to low blood sugar.

What foods is it found in?

- Fruit and vegetables, especially aduki beans, kidney beans and avocados
- Fish and meat

Figures for the glutathione content of food are not available in standard reference works. Glutathione is abundant in many foods but is broken down and inactivated by the digestive system. The glutathione in our bodies is made from the amino acids cysteine, glutamic acid and glycine.

Useful information

Glutathione is depleted by:

- Alcohol consumption
- Cigarette smoking
- Infections
- Over-the-counter medicines such as paracetamol (acetaminophen), especially when combined with alcohol
- Prescription medicines
- Strenuous physical activity.

Many of glutathione's health benefits relate to its role in making the enzyme glutathione peroxidase. This enzyme also needs adequate selenium and zinc. Glutathione levels are extremely depleted in people with chronic illnesses such as chronic fatigue syndrome, Parkinson's disease (linked with pesticide exposure[1]), Aids, cancer, multiple sclerosis and rheumatoid arthritis. People with hyperinsulinaemia—where insulin levels remain permanently high (often due to insulin resistance)—may also develop glutathione deficiency.

In a research study on nine patients with early, untreated Parkinson's disease, intravenous glutathione therapy twice daily for 30 days resulted in a 42 per cent decline in disability. The therapeutic effect lasted for approximately 2-4 months after the end of the treatment period[2].

Paul Cheney MD, who specializes in chronic fatigue syndrome research, finds that glutathione levels are universally low in this condition. He says that low levels of glutathione seem to promote the growth of viruses. By raising the glutathione level, he says, you can stop almost any virus from replicating[3] .

Dr Cheney also points out that if your liver detoxification fails due to low glutathione levels, you become vulnerable to much smaller amounts of toxins. For instance if you have amalgam (silver) fillings—which contain the toxic metal mercury—in your teeth you may begin to suffer from mercury poisoning if you become glutathione-deficient. You can also become vulnerable to poisoning by the normal bacterial toxins produced in your own intestines.

Severe glutathione depletion causes a functional deficiency of folic acid and B12 because these vitamins require glutathione in order to be methylated, or converted to their active form. This creates a vicious circle, as these vitamin deficiencies then lead to further glutathione depletion[4].

There is promising research to suggest that maintaining high glutathione levels may help to extend our natural life span.

SUPPLEMENTS

How to use glutathione supplements

Glutathione can be taken as a dietary supplement, in which case its most effective chemical form is thought to be *reduced* glutathione. But renowned antioxidant researcher Lester Packer does not recommend glutathione supplements, because they may be broken down by digestive enzymes before reaching the body's cells where they are needed. Neither does he recommend n-acetyl cysteine (NAC) supplements although they have been shown to increase glutathione levels. Packer's research suggests that eating foods rich in cysteine, glutamic acid and glycine, plus taking a sister antioxidant known as alpha lipoic acid, is much more effective than glutathione supplements because lipoic acid can quickly and effectively boost the body's own natural glutathione levels by up to 30 per cent. He recommends taking 100 mg of lipoic acid daily for this purpose[5]. He suggests that this can also reverse the slump in immune function which naturally occurs as we get older. Some studies suggest that lipoic acid can even raise glutathione levels by up to 70 per cent[6].

In his work with chronic fatigue syndrome patients, Dr Paul Cheney finds that a lightly denatured whey protein concentrate known as Immunocal has helped many of his patients. Tests showed a steady reduction in lipid peroxides measured in their urine over a period of about six months—a sign that glutathione levels were not only rising, but that body functions dependent on glutathione were improving. Levels of disease-causing bacteria and viruses also gradually reduced to zero.[3] Whey protein concentrate is a good source of cysteine which readily converts to glutathione. Dr Cheney also uses extracts of the herbal medicine milk thistle to help the body regenerate glutathione from its oxidized back to its active (reduced) state. He does not recommend high-dose supplements of n-acetyl cysteine (NAC) for people with chronic fatigue syndrome as they are not well tolerated.

Gluthione can also be increased by taking supplements of s-adenosyl methionine (SAM)[7], green tea[8], vitamin C[9], and the Indian spice turmeric[10].

Nutrients involved in methylation in the body are also essential to keep the body producing glutathione. These include vitamins B6 and B12, folic acid, betaine and the already-mentioned methionine. See page 130 for more information about methylation.

Glycine

What does the body use glycine for?

- Neurotransmitter
- Growth and DNA metabolism
- Forming collagen and phospholipids
- Wound healing
- Blood sugar control
- Energy production
- Making glutathione
- Making bile salts
- Building up glycogen (stored carbohydrate)
- Detoxification of phenols, benzoic acid and other chemicals

Glycine is the simplest of the amino acids, and can be made by the body from the amino acids serine or threonine. It is extremely abundant in the body—almost as abundant as glucose.

Like taurine and GABA it acts as a major inhibitory neurotransmitter, controlling the transmission of electrical impulses along nerves, and is highly concentrated in the brain, particularly in the substantia nigra and hypothalamus—the areas that are subject to degeneration in Parkinson's disease. Glycine is rapidly broken down to serine in the body.

Glycine is a glycogenic amino acid—it is capable of building up glycogen (stored carbohydrate). It assists in the manufacture of DNA, phospholipids (which help substances pass in and out of cells), collagen and glutathione.

Glycine can be converted to pyruvate and thus act as fuel for energy production. It is needed for glycine conjugation—one of the key methods by which the liver breaks down toxins.

Glycine is a potent stimulator for the secretion of glucagon, which controls blood sugar levels. With vitamin B3, chromium, glutamic acid and cysteine, it also forms part of glucose tolerance factor, which helps insulin to function.

Glycine is also essential for wound healing, and, along with zinc, may be added to ointments and creams for this purpose.

What foods is it found in?

- Gelatine
- Almonds, sunflower seeds, peanuts
- Meat, fish
- Buckwheat flour
- Walnuts

19 per cent of the gelatine consists of glycine. Gelatine is a cheap and useful source of this amino acid.

Useful information

People who suffer from gout may benefit from increasing their consumption of glycine-rich foods since this could help their kidneys to break down uric acid more rapidly[1]. Glycine, alanine, aspartic acid and glutamic acid seem to decrease the reabsorption of uric acid by the kidney.

Glycine, in combination with alanine and glutamic acid, has been used to improve the symptoms of an enlarged prostate[2].

Low glycine levels are often found in bipolar and epileptic patients, who may respond to supplementation since glycine is an inhibitory neurotransmitter.

Schizophrenia

Several scientific studies have had encouraging results using glycine supplementation against schizophrenia. In one study, which used a dose of 800 mg glycine per kilo of body weight per day in addition to conventional medication, there was a 30 per cent reduction in symptoms. The lower were the patients' glycine levels before treatment, the better the results[3]. The reason for supplementing glycine is known as the glutamate hypothesis of schizophrenia. According to this theory glutamate is not properly taken up by its receptor sites in some schizophrenics. Glycine binds to the receptors and helps them work more efficiently[4].

Osteoarthritis

People with osteoarthritis treated for 14 weeks with 10 grams of hydrolized gelatine, plus vitamin C and calcium showed significant improvement compared with those on dummy treatments. Those with the most severe symptoms benefited the most. The researchers concluded that gelatine may help enable collagen-forming cells to repair cartilage[5].

Sleep

Glycine plays an important role in normal sleep patterns. Glycine supplementation just prior to bedtime has been shown to improve sleep quality, shortening the latency between sleep onset and initiation of deep sleep. Volunteers also reported less daytime drowsiness and better performance on memory tasks during the day[6].

Dimethylglycine

Dimethylglycine (DMG) is a derivative of the amino acid glycine. It can be found in beans and liver. Like methionine, DMG is a methyl donor. Supplementation with DMG has been suggested for use as an athletic performance enhancer, immunostimulant, and a treatment for autism, epilepsy and mitochondrial disease. For autism, improvement in speech is the most consistent benefit. Behavior and seizures (if present) might also improve[7].

SUPPLEMENTS

How to use glycine supplements

Since glycine is so abundant in foods, there is little point in taking normal commercial supplements, since these would contain less glycine than food itself. The average intake of glycine per day from food is 3-5 grams.

The richest food source of glycine is gelatine, as well as the jelly obtained from boiling skin and bones (for instance chicken carcasses). Although it is not suitable for vegetarians, gelatine can be consumed as a glycine supplement by dissolving it in soup and hot drinks.

How safe are glycine supplements?

The Brain Bio Center in New Jersey has used up to 30 grams a day of glycine in trials without problems[1].

Glycine content of common foods in grams per 100 g

Gelatine, dry	19.05
Almonds, raw	1.47
Sunflower seeds, hulled	1.46
Peanuts, dry roasted	1.43
Beef, ground, extra-lean (approx. 21% fat)	1.31
Prawns, boiled	1.26
Tuna, skipjack, fresh, raw	1.06
Chicken meat, raw	1.05
Pork, composite of various cuts, trimmed, raw	0.98
Buckwheat flour, whole groat	0.98
Salmon, Atlantic, farmed, raw	0.96
Herring, Atlantic, raw	0.86
Oats	0.84
Walnuts, raw	0.82
Brazil nuts, raw	0.66
Wheat flour, whole-grain	0.55
Cheese, cheddar	0.43
Eggs, hard-boiled	0.42
Chick peas, boiled	0.37
Lentils, boiled	0.37
Cornmeal, whole-grain, yellow	0.33
Tofu, raw, with calcium sulphate	0.32
Beans, baked	0.19
Mushrooms, raw	0.13
Rice, brown, long-grain, boiled	0.13
Yoghurt, plain, low-fat	0.13
Broccoli, boiled, drained	0.10
Oranges, raw	0.09
Avocados, raw	0.08
Onions, boiled, drained	0.06
Potatoes, peeled, boiled	0.05
Apricots, raw	0.04
Bananas, raw	0.04
Aubergine (eggplant) boiled, drained	0.03
Beetroot (beets) boiled, drained	0.03
Peppers, sweet, green, raw	0.03
Carrots, boiled, drained	0.03
Cabbage, boiled, drained	0.02
Apples, raw with skin	0.01

Source: USDA National Nutrient Database for Standard Reference, Release 28

Histidine

What does the body use histidine for?

- Making histamine
- Maintenance and growth of tissues
- Copper transport
- As an antioxidant
- Combines with beta-alanine to form the dipeptide carnosine.

Adults and children are able to synthesize histidine from glutamic acid and possibly biotin, but infants (babies) are not. Histidine is an antioxidant which can neutralize the singlet oxygen and hydroxyl free radicals. It is thought to have a mild anti-inflammatory effect because of the way it combines in the blood with copper.

Histidine is used to make histamine, a substance known for its ability to dilate blood vessels and to cause allergic itching and swellings. Histamine also stimulates the secretion of stomach juices and acid, and triggers orgasm when released from mast cells in the genitals.

With the help of folic acid histidine breaks down to form glutamic acid.

What foods is it found in?

- Fish, meat
- Dairy products
- Gelatine

- Peanuts
- Sunflower seeds

Useful information

Research shows that people with rheumatoid arthritis often have low blood histidine levels—possibly due to too-rapid removal of histidine from their blood. Promising results have been achieved by supplementing histidine to these patients, particularly those most seriously affected. Histidine seems to improve their grip strength and walking ability[1] .

Research on rats shows that taking histidine supplements at the same time as non-steroidal anti-inflammatory painkillers such as indomethacin can protect against the gastric inflammation which these drugs are prone to cause[2].

Low plasma concentrations of histidine are associated with wasting, inflammation, oxidative stress, and greater mortality in chronic kidney disease patients. By including L-histidine in an combined amino acid supplement some signs of renal failure can be reversed[3].

Obese women have been found to have lower serum histidine levels and higher levels of inflammation. In a study on obese women with the pre-diabetic condition known as metabolic syndrome, histidine supplementation was found to improve insulin resistance, reduce fat mass and suppress inflammation and oxidative stress. Histidine is thought to improve insulin resistance by reducing the production of pro-inflammatory cytokines and the gene modulator known as NF kappa B[4].

Carnosine

Most of us have heard that cooking foods at high temperatures—especially grilling, barbecuing and deep-frying—produces toxins that are harmful to health. These toxins fall into two categories: benzopyrenes which are known to be carcinogenic, and Advanced Glycation End Products, or AGEs. These are proteins or fats that become glycated as a result of exposure to the sugars found in most foods. AGEs destroy proteins in our body by crosslinking them. They also induce chronic inflammation. Sugar in our blood can react with our own body proteins, forming AGEs which cause the proteins to crosslink. Due to the higher sugar levels in their blood, diabetics are particularly vulnerable to this.

Carnosine, a dipeptide consisting of histidine and beta-alanine, can inhibit glycation and crosslinking, and is considered to have excellent anti-ageing properties[5]. It is available in supplement form, with a suggested dose of 500 mg twice a day.

SUPPLEMENTS

How to use histidine supplements

The suggested dosage for rheumatoid arthritis is four grams a day in divided doses.

How safe are histidine supplements?

Since heavy histamine supplementation may be capable of bringing on a menstrual period, histidine is probably best avoided by women with heavy menstrual bleeding.

According to the work of the late Dr Carl Pfeiffer at the Brain Bio Center in New Jersey, some individuals with clinical depression or schizophrenia have a naturally high histamine level and their illness can be treated by histamine-reducing measures. Since histidine may be able to raise histamine levels, people with mental illness are advised to exercise caution with this supplement.

Histidine content of common foods in grams per 100 g

Cheese, cheddar	0.87
Pork, composite of various cuts, trimmed, raw	0.74
Chicken meat, raw	0.66
Gelatine, dry	0.66
Tuna, skipjack, fresh, raw	0.65
Sunflower seeds, hulled	0.63
Peanuts, dry roasted	0.60
Almonds, raw	0.59
Salmon, Atlantic, farmed, raw	0.59
Beef, ground, extra-lean (approx. 21% fat)	0.56
Herring, Atlantic, raw	0.53
Prawns, boiled	0.43
Oats	0.41
Brazil nuts, raw	0.40
Walnuts, raw	0.39
Wheat flour, whole-grain	0.32
Eggs, hard-boiled	0.30
Buckwheat flour, whole groat	0.29
Lentils, boiled	0.25
Cornmeal, whole-grain, yellow	0.25
Chick peas, boiled	0.24
Tofu, raw, with calcium sulphate	0.24
Beans, baked	0.13
Yoghurt, plain, low-fat	0.13
Bananas, raw	0.08
Mushrooms, raw	0.08
Rice, brown, long-grain, boiled	0.07
Broccoli, boiled, drained	0.05
Potatoes, peeled, boiled	0.04
Avocados, raw	0.03
Apricots, raw	0.03
Beetroot (beets) boiled, drained	0.02
Onions, boiled, drained	0.02
Cabbage, boiled, drained	0.02
Aubergine (eggplant) boiled, drained	0.02
Oranges, raw	0.02
Peppers, sweet, green, raw	0.02
Carrots, boiled, drained	0.02
Apples, raw with skin	0.00

Source: USDA National Nutrient Database for Standard Reference, Release 28

Isoleucine

What does the body use isoleucine for?

- With other branched-chain amino acids, isoleucine is a major component of collagen
- Maintains and stimulates the synthesis of body muscle and other types of protein
- Prevents the breakdown of body proteins in trauma states
- Stimulates the release of alanine from muscle.

Isoleucine is one of the three branched-chain amino acids (BCAAs). The other two are leucine and valine. The BCAAs cannot be made by the human body and must be consumed through food. They are particularly needed by the muscles, and to cope with major stresses such as surgery and severe injuries and infections. They help to prevent hypercatabolism—the breaking down of the body's tissues which can occur after major trauma. If needed for energy, isoleucine can be broken down into two types of fuel: ketones or glucose.

Because of their ability to maintain blood sugar levels, some doctors believe that BCAAs (with other nutrients) may be a more ideal source of energy than glucose in hospital patients who need intravenous feeding, especially as they decrease the rate of breakdown and utilization of other amino acids.

What foods is it found in?

- Cheese
- Gelatine
- Sunflower seeds
- Peanuts
- Meat, fish
- Oats

Useful information

The Brain Bio Center in the US has found that people with chronic schizophrenia may have reduced levels of isoleucine and that supplementation with isoleucine can reverse their illness, especially if given in combination with very large amounts of vitamin B3[1] .

Chronic fatigue syndrome

Research suggests that some patients with chronic fatigue syndrome (also known as ME) may have excessive levels of tryptophan in their plasma. Free tryptophan in the brain is converted to serotonin, which promotes drowsiness and prepares the body for sleep. Persistently high levels of brain serotonin can lead to persistent fatigue.

In severe chronic fatigue syndrome, a small amount of activity leaves the patient feeling as if he/she has done much more. This disease is still very poorly understood, and this symptom may be because the metabolism behaves as if the body has over-exercised. (We know, for instance, that lactic acid levels are often high in chronic fatigue syndrome, whereas in normal individuals they would be high only after much-exertion).

In normal individuals, exertion reduces levels of the branched-chain amino acids, which compete with tryptophan for entry into the brain. This allows larger than usual amounts of tryptophan to enter the brain, where they are converted to serotonin, and promote drowsiness and fatigue. Supplementation with branched-chain amino acids may therefore help to combat excessive tryptophan levels in people with chronic fatigue[2]. It is also important for them to avoid consuming high-carbohydrate meals, which encourage tryptophan uptake into the brain.

SUPPLEMENTS

How to use isoleucine supplements

Isoleucine supplements are usually available only in combined BCAA products.

BCAA supplements are indicated for any form of physical stress and for the healing of severe wounds and injuries. Suggested regimes are 2-4 grams per day of leucine and 1-2 grams each of isoleucine and valine, taken:

- During intensive athletic training
- In chronic fatigue syndrome
- For up to a week before and after participating in a major athletic event
- Plus 1 gram vitamin C and 20 mg zinc, taken as needed after a major injury or fever
- Plus 1 gram vitamin C and 20 mg zinc, taken for up to a week before and two weeks after surgery.

For non-vegetarian athletes, gelatine, which can be stirred into soups and made into jelly with fruit juice, is an ideal supplement as it is cheap and extremely rich in branched-chain amino acids but contains no tryptophan. Other foods rich in BCAAs should also be consumed.

How safe are isoleucine supplements?

BCAAs compete with each other and with tyrosine, phenylalanine, tryptophan and methionine for transport to the brain, so exceptionally high levels of BCAAs (as in intravenous feeding) could lead to a decrease in the brain of the important chemicals serotonin and dopamine, which are made from these amino acids.

Isoleucine content of common foods in grams per 100 g

Cheese, cheddar	1.55
Gelatine, dry	1.16
Sunflower seeds, hulled	1.14
Chicken meat, raw	1.13
Prawns, boiled	1.01
Tuna, skipjack, fresh, raw	1.01
Salmon, Atlantic, farmed, raw	0.92
Pork, composite of various cuts, trimmed, raw	0.87
Peanuts, dry roasted	0.83
Herring, Atlantic, raw	0.83
Beef, ground, extra-lean (approx. 21% fat)	0.76
Oats	0.69
Eggs, hard-boiled	0.69
Almonds, raw	0.69
Walnuts, raw	0.63
Brazil nuts, raw	0.60
Wheat flour, whole-grain	0.51
Buckwheat flour, whole groat	0.47
Tofu, raw, with calcium sulphate	0.40
Lentils, boiled	0.39
Chick peas, boiled	0.38
Cornmeal, whole-grain, yellow	0.29
Yoghurt, plain, low-fat	0.29
Beans, baked	0.21
Broccoli, boiled, drained	0.12
Mushrooms, raw	0.12
Rice, brown, long-grain, boiled	0.11
Avocados, raw	0.07
Potatoes, peeled, boiled	0.07
Cabbage, boiled, drained	0.05
Beetroot (beets) boiled, drained	0.05
Onions, boiled, drained	0.05
Carrots, boiled, drained	0.04
Apricots, raw	0.04
Aubergine (eggplant) boiled, drained	0.04
Bananas, raw	0.03
Peppers, sweet, green, raw	0.03
Oranges, raw	0.03
Apples, raw with skin	0.01

Source: USDA National Nutrient Database for Standard Reference, Release 28

Leucine

What does the body use leucine for?

- With other branched-chain amino acids, leucine is a major component of collagen
- Abundant in ligaments
- Promotes wound healing
- Helps to maintain even blood sugar levels by stimulating the pancreas to release insulin
- Can be used as a source of energy by the muscles instead of glucose.

Leucine is one of the branched-chain amino acids which together make up one third of muscle protein. It cannot be made by the human body and must be consumed through food. Leucine is particularly needed by the muscles, as well as for energy and to cope with major stresses such as surgery and severe injuries and infections. Like fats, leucine is broken down to ketones.

Leucine is especially good at stimulating the body to synthesize protein. Studies show that together with the other branched-chain amino acids (BCAAs) it also helps to prevent hypercatabolism—the breaking down of the body's tissues which can occur after major trauma.

Although several amino acids can be used to produce glucose, leucine is the only amino acid that can be used directly as an energy source instead of glucose when no glucose is available. Because of its ability to maintain blood sugar levels, some doctors believe that leucine (with other nutrients) may be a more ideal source of energy than glucose in hospital patients who need intravenous feeding, particularly as the BCAAs decrease the rate of breakdown and utilization of other amino acids.

BCAAs are used to synthesize the amino acids alanine and glutamine, which can also be converted to glucose.

What foods is it found in?

- Gelatine
- Cheese
- Sunflower seeds
- Meat, fish
- Peanuts and almonds
- Oats

Leucine is more highly concentrated in foods than other amino acids. The body's ability to use leucine is dependent on the presence of adequate B vitamins, copper and magnesium.

Useful information

Leucine is especially useful for marathon runners because it can be used as an energy source when carbohydrate reserves are exhausted.

Although most BCAA research has been carried out on a combination of all the BCAAs, some researchers believe that we should now be emphasizing leucine[1].

Intentional weight loss in the form of a low-calorie diet brings the risk of losing lean tissue as well as fat. Leucine can help prevent this risk[2,3].

Leucine also activates signalling that favourably affects insulin sensitivity and the body's ability to build muscle[4,5].

Body building

While isoleucine and valine are comparatively inefficient for muscle building, leucine is highly metabolically active in promoting muscle tissue synthesis[6].

In a study where 19.7 g of whey protein and 6.2 g leucine were added to the daily diet for 8 weeks, bench-press and push-up performance, total mass, fat-free mass, and lean body mass all increased significantly compared with the placebo (untreated) group[7].

Chronic fatigue syndrome

Research suggests that some patients with chronic fatigue syndrome (also known as ME) may have excessive levels of tryptophan in their plasma. Free tryptophan in the brain is converted to serotonin, which promotes drowsiness and prepares the body for sleep. Persistently high levels of brain serotonin can lead to persistent fatigue[8].

In severe chronic fatigue syndrome, a small amount of activity leaves the patient feeling as if he/she has done much more. This disease is still very poorly understood, and this symptom may be because the metabolism behaves as if the body has over-exercised. (We know, for instance, that lactic acid levels are often high in chronic fatigue syndrome, whereas in normal individuals they would be high only after much exertion).

In normal individuals, exertion reduces levels of the branched-chain amino acids, which compete with tryptophan for entry into the brain. This allows larger than usual amounts of tryptophan to enter the brain, where they are converted to serotonin, and promote drowsiness and fatigue. Supplementation with branched-chain amino acids may therefore help to combat excessive tryptophan levels in chronic fatigue sufferers[9]. It is also important for them to avoid consuming high-carbohydrate meals, which encourage tryptophan uptake into the brain.

SUPPLEMENTS

How to use leucine supplements

A highly-recommended form of BCAA supplement is organic whey protein from grass-fed cows or goats. This is usually purchased in powdered form by the kilo and can be made into a drink. Whey protein is also an excellent way to maximize the body's glutathione levels. Leucine supplements can be added to this, and most users take 1-3 grams twice daily.

BCAA supplements are indicated for any form of physical stress and for the healing of severe wounds and injuries. Consuming them before or during endurance exercise can prevent or reduce the breakdown of muscle protein, help to spare glycogen stores, and improve mental and physical performance[9]. Uses of these supplements include taking them:

- During intensive athletic training
- In chronic fatigue syndrome
- For up to a week before and after participating in a major athletic event
- Plus 1 gram vitamin C and 20 mg zinc, taken as needed after a major injury or fever
- Plus 1 gram vitamin C and 20 mg zinc, taken for up to a week before and two weeks after surgery.

Gelatine, which can be stirred into soups and made into jelly with fruit juice, may be a good supplement for those with chronic fatigue syndrome as it is cheap and extremely rich in branched-chain amino acids but contains no tryptophan.

How safe are leucine supplements?

BCAAs compete with each other and with tyrosine, phenylalanine, tryptophan and methionine for transport to the brain, so exceptionally high levels of BCAAs (as in intravenous feeding) could lead to a decrease in the brain of the important chemicals serotonin and dopamine, which are made from these amino acids. High levels of leucine also seem to increase the excretion of vitamin B3 in the urine.

The presence of large amounts of leucine can reduce the availability of nitric oxide (NO) in the blood vessels. Low NO levels can encourage insulin resistance[10].

Some researchers propose an upper level of 0.53 grams per kilo of body weight per day as a safe upper limit of leucine intake[11].

Leucine content of common foods in grams per 100 g

Gelatine, dry	2.45
Cheese, cheddar	2.39
Tuna, skipjack, fresh, raw	1.79
Sunflower seeds, hulled	1.66
Prawns, boiled	1.66
Salmon, Atlantic, farmed, raw	1.62
Chicken meat, raw	1.61
Peanuts, dry roasted	1.54
Pork, composite of various cuts, trimmed, raw	1.51
Almonds, raw	1.47
Herring, Atlantic, raw	1.46
Beef, ground, extra-lean (approx. 21% fat)	1.42
Oats	1.28
Brazil nuts, raw	1.19
Walnuts, raw	1.17
Eggs, hard-boiled	1.08
Cornmeal, whole-grain, yellow	1.00
Wheat flour, whole-grain	0.93
Buckwheat flour, whole groat	0.79
Lentils, boiled	0.65
Chick peas, boiled	0.63
Tofu, raw, with calcium sulphate	0.61
Yoghurt, plain, low-fat	0.53
Beans, baked	0.38
Rice, brown, long-grain, boiled	0.21
Mushrooms, raw	0.18
Broccoli, boiled, drained	0.14
Avocados, raw	0.12
Potatoes, peeled, boiled	0.10
Apricots, raw	0.08
Bananas, raw	0.07
Beetroot (beets) boiled, drained	0.07
Aubergine (eggplant) boiled, drained	0.05
Cabbage, boiled, drained	0.05
Onions, boiled, drained	0.05
Carrots, boiled, drained	0.05
Peppers, sweet, green, raw	0.05
Oranges, raw	0.02
Apples, raw with skin	0.01

Source: USDA National Nutrient Database for Standard Reference, Release 28

Lysine

What does the body use lysine for?

- Synthesis of hormones, antibodies and enzymes
- Regulates calcium absorption
- Collagen production (using vitamin C and iron)
- Carnitine production
- Production of the amino acids citrulline and homoarginine (needed for protein metabolism)
- Production of the neurotransmitter pipecolic acid

Lysine cannot be made by the body and must be obtained from the diet. It is highly concentrated in the muscles, and is primarily metabolized to acetyl CoA, a critical nutrient in energy production. Lysine is also used to make carnitine, an important amino acid for the conversion of fat to energy. Carnitine can be obtained either from the diet (meat or dairy products) or through synthesis in the body using lysine and vitamin B6.

The body's ability to break down lysine depends on vitamins B2 and B3.

What foods is it found in?

- Dairy products
- Meat, fish
- Tofu
- Beans and lentils
- Broccoli
- Potatoes

Kidney stones

The number one cause of kidney stones is not drinking enough water. However lysine may be a natural regulator of calcium oxalate in urine, helping to prevent crystallization which may lead to oxalate kidney stone formation[1].

Osteoporosis

Calcium deficiency contributes to age-related bone loss (osteoporosis). Studies have shown that L-lysine supplements can increase the absorption of calcium from food in the intestines and reduce calcium losses in the urine. This may be of value against osteoporosis[2].

Herpes infections

Eating a diet which emphasizes lysine at the expense of the amino acid arginine seems to be able to help people suffering from viruses belonging to the herpes family. On the other hand diets which emphasize arginine at the expense of lysine seem to encourage the growth of these viruses. People who suffer from recurrent herpes virus sores such as genital herpes or cold sores have reported that taking lysine supplements helps them more than any other treatments[3]. Lysine and arginine share the same transport system in the body. Lysine supplementation results in the system having a smaller capacity to absorb and distribute arginine.

In one research study, the rate of herpes infections was 2.4 times less when lysine supplements (one gram three times a day) were taken, compared with the group on the placebo (dummy) treatment. Symptoms and healing time were considerably reduced[4]. Research studies using smaller doses do not seem to work, although this may perhaps be due to not prescribing a low-arginine diet.

Chronic fatigue syndrome and ME

People suffering from chronic fatigue syndrome are often infected with the Epstein-Barr virus, which is a member of the herpes virus family (see Herpes infections above). If you have chronic fatigue it makes sense to keep to a diet with a low arginine to lysine ratio (see table on page 126).

Anxiety

In a double-blind, placebo controlled, randomized study, 108 subjects were given either a week-long oral treatment with L-lysine (2.64 g per day) and L-arginine (2.64 g per day) or placebo. The treated group showed significantly reduced general anxiety, stress-induced anxiety, and basal levels of stress hormones[5].

After a systematic review, it was concluded that there is strong evidence for the use of herbal supplements containing extracts of passionflower or kava and combinations of L-lysine and L-arginine as treatments for anxiety symptoms and disorders[6].

Heart disease

The late Linus Pauling PhD was a strong advocate of taking lysine supplements together with vitamin C to reduce atherosclerosis—deposits of cholesterol on artery walls resulting in narrowed arteries and heart disease. The rationale for this treatment is as follows:

- Nutritional deficiencies, especially of vitamin C and flavonoids, cause structural weaknesses to develop in artery walls.
- The body attempts to repair them, by incorporating fatty particles of lipoprotein (a) into artery walls.
- This attracts cholesterol deposits, which form on the inside of the artery walls, leading to narrowed arteries and heart disease.

Lysine can make lipoprotein particles slippery, forcing them to detach from the blood vessel wall, thus dislodging the cholesterol deposits. Large quantities of supplementary lysine need to be consumed to achieve this effect. At the same time the vitamin C deficiency needs to be corrected, to promote the good health of vessel walls[7].

SUPPLEMENTS

How to use lysine supplements

Herpes

Lysine supplements are extensively used to treat herpes virus infections. If taken in conjunction with zinc and vitamin C supplements, and a high-lysine low-arginine diet, 1-3 grams of lysine three times a day is thought to be enough to reduce symptoms and shorten healing time if a flare-up occurs. To prevent recurrences, a typical dose is one gram, 1-3 times a day. Take lysine supplements on their own, away from protein and other amino acid supplements, especially arginine and cysteine.

(Continued on page 128)

Arginine to lysine ratio in common foods	Lysine g/100g	Arginine g/100g	Ratio
Walnuts, raw	0.42	2.28	5.4
Brazil nuts, raw	0.54	2.39	4.4
Almonds, raw	0.60	2.47	4.1
Coconut meat, raw	0.15	0.55	3.7
Peanuts, dry roasted	0.85	2.83	3.3
Onions, boiled, drained	0.07	0.18	2.8
Sunflower seeds, hulled	0.94	2.40	2.6
Rice, brown, long-grain, boiled	0.10	0.20	2.0
Gelatine, dry	3.46	6.62	1.9
Millet, boiled	0.07	0.12	1.8
Cornmeal, whole-grain, yellow	0.23	0.41	1.8
Oats	0.70	1.19	1.7
Wheat flour, whole-grain	0.38	0.64	1.7
Buckwheat flour, whole groat	0.64	0.94	1.5
Chick peas, boiled	0.59	0.84	1.4
Oranges, raw	0.05	0.07	1.4
Peas, green, boiled, drained	0.31	0.42	1.3
Cabbage, boiled, drained	0.05	0.06	1.2
Aubergine (eggplant) boiled, drained	0.04	0.05	1.2
Dark chocolate	0.21	0.24	1.1
Cocoa powder, dry	0.98	1.11	1.1
Lentils, boiled	0.63	0.70	1.1
Peppers, sweet, green, raw	0.04	0.04	1.1
Carrots, boiled, drained	0.04	0.05	1.0
Broccoli, boiled, drained	0.15	0.16	1.0
Tofu, raw, with calcium sulphate	0.53	0.54	1.0
Mung beans, boiled, drained	0.49	0.49	1.0
Prawns, boiled	1.82	1.83	1.0
Pumpkin, boiled, drained	0.04	0.04	1.0
Bananas, raw	0.05	0.05	1.0
Butter beans (lima beans), boiled,	0.52	0.48	0.9
Beans, baked	0.33	0.30	0.9
Beef, ground, extra lean (21% fat)	1.48	1.19	0.8
Eggs, hard-boiled	0.90	0.76	0.8
Potatoes, peeled, boiled	0.10	0.08	0.8
Beetroot (beets) boiled, drained	0.06	0.04	0.7
Chicken meat, raw	1.82	1.29	0.7
Pork, composite of various cuts,	1.70	1.20	0.7
Salmon, Atlantic, farmed, raw	1.83	1.19	0.7
Herring, Atlantic, raw	1.65	1.08	0.7

Tuna, skipjack, fresh, raw	2.02	1.32	0.7
Avocados, raw	0.09	0.06	0.6
Apples, raw with skin	0.01	0.01	0.5
Mushrooms, raw	0.29	0.14	0.5
Milk chocolate	0.41	0.20	0.5
Apricots, raw	0.10	0.05	0.5
Cheese, cheddar	2.07	0.94	0.5
Yoghurt, plain, low-fat	0.47	0.16	0.3

Source: USDA National Nutrient Database for Standard Reference, Release 28

Notes

If you are combating herpes virus, shingles or Epstein-Barr, avoid the highlighted foods unless eating them in negligible amounts, since these foods have both a high arginine:lysine ratio (more than 1.0) and a high arginine content. The remaining foods are acceptable either because

- (E.g. rice) normal consumption will not result in a significant arginine intake,
- Or the arginine content is balanced by lysine,
- Or (e.g. cocoa powder) the foods are unlikely to be consumed in significant quantities.

To date, advice on balancing lysine and arginine through diet has been scanty and unreliable. For instance most publications advise the avoidance of chocolate when in fact milk chocolate has a low arginine ratio and even pure cocoa only has a ratio of 1.1. Much more relevant as a potential problem is gelatine, used in many desserts and confectionery products. A handful of dry gelatine powder can yield as much as 6.6 grams of arginine, and has a high ratio at 1.9. Most other grains, nuts and seeds which are not mentioned on the list also have a high arginine:lysine ratio.

Atherosclerosis

Dr Linus Pauling's recommendations were as follows:
500 mg vitamin C together with 1 gram L-lysine, three times daily on an empty stomach between meals. Double this dose after two weeks and ask your doctor to monitor your lipoprotein (a) levels.

How safe are lysine supplements?

Supplementation with more than 2 grams of lysine per day may reduce the activity of the enzyme arginase, which is needed to break down toxic ammonia into urea. Excessive lysine supplementation can also raise blood cholesterol and triglyceride (fat) levels.

Methionine and
S-adenosyl-methionine (SAM)

What does the body use methionine for?

- As a primary methyl donor
- To make cysteine and taurine
- For creatine, phosphatidylcholine and glutathione synthesis
- To make enkephalins and endorphins
- To metabolize homocysteine and serine
- Combines with toxins to allow them to be eliminated
- Helps to remove excess oestrogen, adrenaline, histamine and related substances
- Contributes to the health of neurons and joints.

Methionine is one of the sulphur amino acids. It cannot be synthesized by the human body, and must be obtained from the diet. It is vital for the synthesis of other sulphur amino acids (cysteine and taurine), and donates sulphur and other compounds required to make many other substances. Without a sufficient daily intake of methionine the body cannot produce adequate adrenaline and other hormones.

Methionine is a component of the body's natural painkillers enkephalin and endorphin, and has sometimes been used as a painkilling treatment. It is also essential in regulating the availability of folic acid. A methionine-deficient diet can cause folic acid deficiency as this B vitamin becomes trapped in the liver in an inactive form—

hence recent research into its use against spina bifida, where previously only folic acid supplementation was used as a preventive measure.

Environmental medicine expert Dr William Rea says that in people with degenerative diseases, mental illness or food and chemical allergies, methionine is the most disrupted of all their body's amino acids[1].

What foods is it found in?

- Brazil nuts
- Meat, fish
- Sunflower and sesame seeds
- Dairy products
- Oats

Vegans should take special care to obtain enough methionine. Beans and most soy products are poor sources of this amino acid.

Methylation and homocysteine

When methionine reacts with the body's energy source known as ATP it forms s-adenosyl-methionine (SAM or SAMe), sometimes known as 'activated' methionine. Methionine is mostly used in this form. SAM donates methyl groups or CH3—a carbon atom attached to three hydrogen atoms—to help break down toxins and excesses of hormones such as adrenaline and oestrogen, and for the synthesis of a host of important biological compounds, including betaine, carnitine, choline, creatine, adrenal hormones, melatonin and nucleic acids. The donation process is known as methylation. Methylation is involved in maintaining DNA integrity, processing fats, improving neurological function, liver detoxification, and is connected to nearly every biochemical process in the body. Poor methylation is linked to a large variety of age-related diseases.

In order to metabolize (use) methionine, the body requires adequate amounts of B vitamins (especially folic acid and B12), magnesium and serine. If a diet high in methionine is consumed but the methionine is not properly metabolized, there is a risk of homocysteine levels rising. Psychiatric and nervous system problems can also develop when insufficient methionine is converted to SAM.

Raised homocysteine levels in the blood have become an easily definable sign of poor methylation. Along with other methyl donors vitamin B6, B12, folate and betaine, methionine is essential for the metabolism of homocysteine. If allowed to build up in the blood, homocysteine can encourage a harmful build-up of cholesterol deposits in arteries and recent research is linking it with the development of an increasing number of diseases, notably Alzheimer's disease and osteoporosis, as well as poor liver detoxification. Symptoms of poor detoxification are many and varied, and include headaches and chronic fatigue.

Allergies and histamine

Studies on rats suggest that methionine supplementation may be able to increase levels of adrenal hormones in the body. This may be one reason why Dr Eric Braverman, formerly of the Brain Bio Center in New Jersey, and author of the *Healing Nutrients Within,* describes methionine as a good allergy fighter. The body tries to combat allergic inflammation by producing adrenal hormones such as cortisol. The other reason is methionine's ability to reduce high levels of histamine—a substance responsible for allergic inflammation and swellings.

Schizophrenia

The Brain Bio Center in the USA uses methionine to treat one type of schizophrenia, classified as the 'high histamine' type, which is associated with severe depression and suicidal tendencies. The Brain Bio Center believes that L-methionine alleviates depression by lowering blood histamine[2]. Others (using SAM supplements) believe it may work by increasing the turnover of the mood-governing substances noradrenaline, dopamine and serotonin[3]. On the other hand excessive supplementation with methionine can aggravate psychotic symptoms in other types of schizophrenia where individuals suffer from folic acid deficiency[2].

Many drugs used in psychiatric medicine work by keeping up the body's levels of adrenal hormones. It is not surprising that similar effects can be achieved by increasing consumption of the raw materials which the body uses to make these hormones.

Depression

Despite the availability of a large array of pharmaceutical antidepressants, many patients continue to experience a relatively modest response while suffering a burden of side effects. A review of recent research into the use of folic acid and SAM supplements in mood disorders suggests that supplementation with SAM and methylfolate (the methylated or 'active' form of folic acid) appear to be efficacious and well tolerated in reducing depression symptoms[4].

For several decades researchers have been claiming that SAM yields results comparable to those of conventional treatments[5,6]. Some researchers describe SAM as a very effective antidepressant, with a more rapid therapeutic effect than that of standard tricyclic antidepressants, which makes it very beneficial for those in a catatonic state or those with acute suicidal thoughts[5].

Alzheimer's disease

Alzheimer's disease is accompanied by diminished glutathione and SAM, and increased homocysteine. Recent findings confirm that SAM can directly boost glutathione activity.

One of the most important nutrients for Alzheimer's patients is choline, first because it is needed for the memory neurotransmitter acetylcholine, and second because it is used to make betaine, a substance recently found to be just as important to break down homocysteine as vitamins B6, B12 and folic acid[7]. SAM supplements can help to maintain the availability of both choline and acetylcholine and can restore cognitive performance to normal levels after acetylcholine deficiency[8].

SAM supplements have also been found to improve mental function, mood and speed of mental processing in patients with Alzheimer's disease[9].

Researchers conclude that SAM is extremely important in the maintenance of neuron (nerve cell) health and suggest that SAM supplements should be used in the treatment of Alzheimer's disease[10,11,12].

Motor neurone disease (ALS)

Oxidative stress is recognized as a contributing factor to motor neurone disease (also known as ALS). In animal studies, mice bred to display changes characteristic of ALS were supplemented with SAM. The onset of the disease was delayed by 2-3 weeks compared with unsupplemented mice. SAM also delayed hallmarks of neurodegeneration in these mice, including preventing loss of motor neurons. Unfortunately SAM was not able to increase their survival time[13].

Drug toxicity

Methotrexate is a drug used in low doses to treat rheumatoid arthritis. Research has raised concerns about its abilitiy to disrupt methylation, which could bring many harmful consequences. Methylation is involved in maintaining DNA integrity, processing fats, improving nerve function, liver detoxification, and is connected to nearly every biochemical process in the body. Poor methylation is linked to a large variety of diseases. The researchers believe that supplementation with SAM would help to compensate for this side effect of the drug[14].

Liver toxicity caused by cancer chemotherapy can cause much disruption to chemotherapy regimes. Because glutathione helps to protect the liver, and SAM supplements can raise liver glutathione levels, some researchers have administered SAM supplements to cancer patients who developed chemotherapy-induced liver toxicity. Signs of toxicity were significantly reduced after 1-2 weeks of SAM therapy. The beneficial effects persisted, allowing the patients to continue their chemotherapy with minimum disruption[15].

Migraine

Long-term SAM supplementation has been found to relieve pain in migraine sufferers. The benefit arises gradually and long-term treatment is required for therapeutic effectiveness[16].

Liver function

SAM supplementation is known to restore liver glutathione and to reduce liver injury. A meta-analysis of recent research provides positive evidence that SAM supplements are useful to include in a regime for liver function improvement though they do not help some types of chronic liver disease[17,18].

Spina bifida

Neural tube defects (NTD) are a type of birth defect resulting in the incomplete development, or even the absence of the brain and spinal cord. Spina bifida is an example of this type of defect. In a five-year study on 170 pregnancies with neural tube defects a 30-55% lower risk of NTD was found among the women with the highest average daily intakes of methionine[19]. Although folic acid deficiency is normally associated with NTD, methionine is required to convert folic acid into its active form.

Other uses of SAM supplementation include:
- Increasing the body's production of phosphatidyl-choline[17], which can improve the flexibility of red blood cells, helping them squeeze through narrow capillaries and supply more oxygen to tissues.

- Enhancing the synthesis of cartilage-building proteoglycans in people with osteoarthritis. SAM is an important component of joint tissue, and SAM supplementation has been evaluated in more than 22,000 osteoarthritis patients. The symptoms usually improve after two weeks of supplementation[17].
- Improving pain and morning stiffness in patients with fibromyalgia (muscle pain associated with chronic fatigue syndrome)[17].
- Researchers have also used SAM supplements to combat parkinsonism[3,20,21]. SAM is needed for the vital process of converting L-DOPA to dopamine and is often depleted in patients with Parkinson's disease.

SUPPLEMENTS

How to use methionine supplements

The suggested dosage of SAM is 200-800 mg am and pm, with a maintenance dose of 200 mg per day once the maximum improvement has been obtained.

How safe are methionine supplements?

Researchers have used up to 5 grams a day of L-methionine against parkinsonism, and up to 2 grams a day against pancreatitis.

SAM supplements may worsen Parkinson's disease, whereas this problem does not seem to occur with normal L-methionine supplements. SAM supplements sometimes cause digestive discomfort such as nausea, vomiting and dry mouth[5,8].

Methionine content of common foods in grams per 100 g

Brazil nuts, raw	1.01
Cheese, cheddar	0.65
Tuna, skipjack, fresh, raw	0.65
Gelatine, dry	0.61
Chicken meat, raw	0.59
Prawns, boiled	0.59
Salmon, Atlantic, farmed, raw	0.59
Herring, Atlantic, raw	0.53
Sunflower seeds, hulled	0.49
Pork, composite of various cuts, trimmed, raw	0.49
Beef, ground, extra-lean (approx. 21% fat)	0.41
Eggs, hard-boiled	0.39
Oats	0.31
Peanuts, dry roasted	0.29
Walnuts, raw	0.24
Wheat flour, whole-grain	0.21
Almonds, raw	0.19
Cornmeal, whole-grain, yellow	0.17
Buckwheat flour, whole groat	0.16
Yoghurt, plain, low-fat	0.16
Chick peas, boiled	0.12
Tofu, raw, with calcium sulphate	0.10
Lentils, boiled	0.08
Beans, baked	0.07
Rice, brown, long-grain, boiled	0.06
Mushrooms, raw	0.06
Avocados, raw	0.04
Broccoli, boiled, drained	0.04
Potatoes, peeled, boiled	0.03
Oranges, raw	0.02
Beetroot (beets) boiled, drained	0.02
Bananas, raw	0.01
Onions, boiled, drained	0.01
Peppers, sweet, green, raw	0.01
Cabbage, boiled, drained	0.01
Aubergine (eggplant) boiled, drained	0.01
Carrots, boiled, drained	0.01
Apricots, raw	0.01
Apples, raw with skin	0.00

Source: USDA National Nutrient Database for Standard Reference, Release 28

Ornithine

What does the body use ornithine for?

- Helping to remove excess ammonia
- Precursor to citrulline, proline and glutamic acid
- Wound healing and immune system benefits (by boosting arginine levels)
- Other similar effects to arginine

Ornithine is not incorporated into proteins in the body. It is involved in the urea cycle, which breaks down the toxin ammonia, allowing it to be excreted in the urine and at the same time arginine is created. So ornithine is also considered as a precursor to arginine.

Ornithine produces the same benefits as arginine, but is thought to be more effective because it enters the cell whereas arginine does not.

What foods is it found in?

- Meat and fish (especially clams and tuna)
- Cheese
- Eggs

Figures for the ornithine content of foods are not yet available in standard amino acid reference works. The western diet typically provides about 5 grams a day of ornithine.

Useful information

Ammonia levels in the blood rise in the presence of liver disease or after prolonged exercise. Due to its ability to remove ammonia, ornithine is used as a drug therapy for people with cirrhosis of the liver, and can also improve the feeling of fatigue in patients with liver disease or after prolonged exercise. People who are sensitive to alcohol may find that taking ornithine supplements before drinking can help to reduce flushing and hangover[1].

Research using one form of ornithine known as ornithine alpha-ketoglutarate on people hospitalized for surgery, trauma or burns, has shown several beneficial effects, including improvement in appetite, weight gain and shorter recovery periods[2].

The presence of large amounts of the amino acid lysine in the body can prevent the uptake of both ornithine and arginine.

Body-building

Owing to one or two research studies, ornithine has gained a reputation of being able to stimulate the production of growth hormone if taken in very large amounts—more than five grams a day. Many body-builders are taking ornithine supplements in the hope of gaining this benefit. In a recent clinical trial, arginine and ornithine were supplemented to athletes during a 3-week heavy resistance training programme. In the supplemented group, significant increases in the serum levels of growth hormone and insulin-like growth factor were found in measurements taken after two minutes and one hour of training[3].

Stress

Based on results obtained from animal studies, researchers tested L-ornithine supplements for their ability to relieve stress and improve sleep and fatigue symptoms in humans. In a randomized, double-blind, placebo-controlled clinical study, fifty-two healthy adults who had previously felt slight stress and fatigue were randomly assigned to either the L-ornithine (400 mg/day) or placebo group. After eight weeks serum levels of the stress hormone cortisol were significantly decreased in the L-ornithine group, anger was reduced and perceived sleep quality had improved[4].

SUPPLEMENTS

How to use ornithine supplements

Many people take ornithine (together with arginine) as a body-building supplement. There is some evidence that these supplements may stimulate the release of growth hormone and insulin, and so increase muscle bulk. In fact Dr Eric Braverman, author of the *Healing Nutrients Within,* suggests that ornithine is a better arginine supplement than arginine itself, because it enters the mitochondria (the energy-producing part of the cell) more readily than arginine. The body readily converts ornithine to arginine. Most scientists doubt that these two amino acids really can have a significant effect, because the research is scanty. Some researchers say that very large doses are necessary to achieve any effect at all, but results from other research say that increases in lean body mass and strength can be achieved with just one gram a day of each amino acid[5].

The suggested dosage for body-building is 500 mg of arginine and 500 mg of ornithine twice a day on an empty stomach, five days a week in combination with weight training.

How safe are ornithine supplements?

Dr Eric Braverman points out that ornithine is associated with an increase in polyamines—substances which may contribute to the growth of cancerous cells. While no harmful effects have been reported from ornithine supplementation, it is probably not advisable to take more than 10 grams a day simply because there is no research into possible adverse effects at this level. In one study using 13 grams a day to increase growth hormone levels, there were many digestive side effects. Dr Braverman has found that doses as low as 1 gram per day may cause insomnia in some individuals[6].

Long-term (exceeding a few years) supplementation and high concentrations (exceeding 600 µmol/l) of ornithine in the blood have been found to cause toxicity to the retina of the eye.

L-Phenylalanine and DL-phenylalanine (DLPA)

What does the body use phenylalanine for?

- To make tyrosine, which in turn is converted to a number of other hormones
- To make cholecystokinin, which is involved in appetite control
- To make phenylethylamine, a mood-elevating substance found in the brain.

Phenylalanine cannot be synthesized by the body, and must be obtained from the diet. It is highly concentrated in the brain, and a deficiency can lead to a wide variety of changes in behaviour. The body's ability to utilize phenylalanine depends on adequate levels of iron, vitamins B3, B6 and C and copper, plus a form of folic acid known as biopterin.

Phenylalanine is the raw material of the important amino acid tyrosine which in turn gives rise to the hormones dopamine, adrenaline (epinephrine in the U.S.), noradrenaline (norepinephrine) and thyroxine. These hormones are involved in a wide range of functions, including blood sugar and blood pressure control, mood and mental alertness, control of the body's movements, and its ability to cope with stress.

What foods is it found in?

- Gelatine
- Cheese
- Peanuts
- Sunflower seeds
- Almonds
- Oats

The average diet provides about 5 grams a day of phenylalanine.

Useful information

Chronically low phenylalanine or tyrosine levels can lead to depression and hypothyroidism, due to a lack of the adrenal hormones and thyroid hormones which are dependent on these amino acids[1].

When phenylalanine is synthesized in the laboratory, it emerges in two forms, known as the D and L isomers. The D isomer of amino acids is not usually found in nature and is not normally utilizable by the human body. But phenylalanine appears to be an exception. A combination of D-phenylalanine and L-phenylalanine (known as DLPA) does seem to have some therapeutic value as a natural painkiller[2]. It is thought to work by preventing the breakdown of the body's own natural painkillers, the endorphins and enkephalins, which are produced by the brain and resemble morphine[3].

Pain

DLPA concentrates selectively on chronic, useless pain, such as:

- Arthritis
- Whiplash
- Low back pain

and is claimed to be effective in 80-95% of users[4]. Users report that DLPA is not toxic, not addictive, does not become less effective in time, and pain relief can last far beyond the period in which DLPA is taken. DLPA normally takes one to three weeks to start controlling pain. Physicians who have prescribed DLPA together with opiate type painkillers find that this combination may amplify pain relief and also ease depression[5].

Appetite control

Phenylalanine can also be used for appetite control. It stimulates the release of an appetite-suppressing hormone called cholecystokinin (CCK) from the wall of the small intestine, which is normally released when food has been consumed. In a clinical trial, six normal-weight subjects were administered 10 grams of L-phenylalanine or placebo (a dummy substance) and a test meal was given to coincide with the peak plasma concentrations of CCK which normally occur 20 minutes after taking phenylalanine. Hunger, desire to eat, and fullness assessments were made before and at several intervals after the meal. The subjects consumed an average of 1,089 Calories after phenylalanine, compared with 1,587 after the placebo. Despite eating less, those who had taken phenylalanine had a greater sensation of fullness[6].

Addiction

Eighteen days of D-phenylananine supplementation can turn mice bred as alcoholics into mice who do not like alcohol at all[7]. This effect is attributed to DLPA's ability to inhibit enzymes which break down the body's natural endorphins. We now know that endorphins and the neurotransmitter dopamine play an enormous role in addictive behaviour of all types.

In recent years, scientists have learned much about the biochemistry of addiction. What was once thought to be the 'addiction gene' is now known as the 'reward deficiency' gene. This gene is mostly found in individuals with various impulsive, compulsive, obsessive and addictive disorders including alcoholism, illegal drug-taking, excessive gambling, morbid obesity and thrill-seeking behaviours ranging all the way from high-risk sports to pathological violence. The temporary feelings of satisfaction experienced as a result of these activities are the 'reward'.

The brain chemistry involved in the reward sensation begins with the release of serotonin, which in turn stimulates endorphins, which in turn inhibit GABA, which in turn fine-tunes the amount of dopamine released at the brain's 'reward site'. The reward sensation occurs as dopamine interacts with dopamine receptors.

In most individuals, the feel-good or reward sensation is triggered by day-to-day pleasurable events. But people who carry the reward deficiency gene have a biological problem known as 'dopamine resistance'. Just as insulin resistance means insulin doesn't work properly and more and more insulin is required before sugar can be removed from our blood, dopamine resistance means that the individual needs more and more dopamine to experience any feelings of well-being. This drives the individual towards dopamine stimulants, or more extreme reward-seeking behaviour. Opiate (narcotic) drugs such as heroin, methadone and morphine massively raise levels of endorphins and dopamine. But over time, the body starts requiring more and more of the opiate to achieve the same high. That is known as drug tolerance. Soon the body becomes dependent on opiates; it stops making endorphins and dopamine without them.

When an opiate abuser lowers his dosage or comes off the drugs completely, s/he experiences a massive endorphin and dopamine deficiency, bringing heightened sensitivity to physical and emotional pain, inability to experience pleasure, and no drive or desire to get anything done. Life basically sucks. This is why opiate abusers so often relapse after quitting drugs. It feels like the only way to experience pleasure is to start using them again.

Phenylalanine in the form DLPA, together with L-tyrosine and 5-HTP are some of the main ingredients in a new patented product known as KB220Z which has been used in more than 20 studies to treat Reward Deficiency Sydrome, which is now the medical term for addictive behaviour[8]. DLPA helps to keep up levels of endorphins by preventing their break-down. It also raises dopamine. L-tyrosine helps to make dopamine. 5-HTP raises serotonin. Scientists hope that this product will reverse the abnormal brain chemistry which causes Reward Deficiency Syndrome.

There is still much research work to be done, but meanwhile, the Opiate Addiction Support website: http://opiateaddictionsupport.com offers a protocol for the use of DLPA supplements to help with opiate withdrawal. They recommend starting DLPA at a high dose while gradually tapering off the opiates and finally tapering off the DLPA dose. A high proportion of recovering addicts visiting this site report that the protocol has been extremely effective for them.

Other uses

Clinical trials have shown that supplements of phenylalanine, or its metabolite tyrosine can be as effective as the antidepressant drug imipramine in people suffering from clinical depression[9].

Another use for phenylalanine supplements is in the treatment of vitiligo, a condition where patches of skin have no pigment and do not tan. In a study where subjects took 50 mg phenylalanine per kilo of their body weight, followed 30-45 minutes later (when blood phenylalanine concentrations were at their peak) by ultra-violet lamp treatment, reasonable pigmentation was obtained after 32 treatments. The patients were able to tolerate more sun than usual, and they experienced no sunburn as a result of the therapy[10].

SUPPLEMENTS

How to use phenylalanine supplements

Pain relief

Begin by taking 1,000 mg DLPA before each meal until significant pain relief occurs. If this does not happen within three weeks, double the dose and try again for another three weeks. If DLPA works for you, the dosage can be decreased once pain relief is obtained. Ensure that your intake of vitamins C and B6 is adequate.

Appetite control

Take 500 mg L-phenylalanine 20 minutes before each meal.

Opiate withdrawal

Start with 1000 to 2000 mg DLPA 3 times per day while gradually tapering off opiates. Slowly reduce the dose once drug withdrawal is complete.

How safe are phenylalanine supplements?

Excessive phenylalanine can cause anxiety, headaches and high blood pressure. These supplements are best avoided by women who are pregnant or breast-feeding. DLPA supplements are widely regarded as very safe. But there are many doubts about the safety of aspartame, the artificial sweetener which contains phenylalanine as one of its ingredients. Many symptoms have been reported from its consumption, including:

- Headaches
- Dizziness
- Fatigue and weakness
- Skin rash
- Tummy pains
- Vomiting and nausea
- Sleep problems

Aspartame (also known as Nutrasweet and Canderel) is found in diet drinks and low-calorie desserts such as yoghurt and ice cream. It is also sold in tablets and granules for adding to food and drinks.

Individuals diagnosed with phenylketonuria (PKU) must not take any form of phenylalanine supplement. PKU is a serious health problem in which, due to a defective gene, the individual cannot metabolize phenylalanine, and becomes severely retarded, with an IQ often of less than 20. Phenylalanine levels can rise to 400 times the normal level. PKU sufferers have especially high needs for vitamin B6. The treatment for this disease is a low-phenylalanine diet.

Phenylalanine content of common foods in grams/100 g

Gelatine, dry	1.74
Cheese, cheddar	1.31
Peanuts, dry roasted	1.23
Sunflower seeds, hulled	1.17
Almonds, raw	1.15
Oats	0.90
Prawns, boiled	0.88
Tuna, skipjack, fresh, raw	0.86
Chicken meat, raw	0.85
Salmon, Atlantic, farmed, raw	0.78
Pork, composite of various cuts, trimmed, raw	0.75
Brazil nuts, raw	0.75
Walnuts, raw	0.71
Herring, Atlantic, raw	0.70
Beef, ground, extra-lean (approx. 21% fat)	0.67
Eggs, hard-boiled	0.67
Wheat flour, whole-grain	0.65
Buckwheat flour, whole groat	0.50
Chick peas, boiled	0.48
Lentils, boiled	0.45
Cornmeal, whole-grain, yellow	0.40
Tofu, raw, with calcium sulphate	0.39
Yoghurt, plain, low-fat	0.29
Beans, baked	0.26
Rice, brown, long-grain, boiled	0.13
Mushrooms, raw	0.11
Broccoli, boiled, drained	0.09
Potatoes, peeled, boiled	0.08
Avocados, raw	0.07
Apricots, raw	0.05
Beetroot (beets) boiled, drained	0.05
Bananas, raw	0.04
Aubergine (eggplant) boiled, drained	0.04
Onions, boiled, drained	0.04
Carrots, boiled, drained	0.03
Cabbage, boiled, drained	0.03
Oranges, raw	0.03
Peppers, sweet, green, raw	0.03
Apples, raw with skin	0.01

Source: USDA National Nutrient Database for Standard Reference, Release 28

Proline

What does the body use proline for?

- Major constituent of collagen
- Allows proteins to have a sharp bend or turn in their shape
- Wound healing

Proline can be made from either glutamic acid or ornithine in the human body. It is also found in food. Its main role is in collagen maintenance and repair. (Collagen is a protein which helps to form the structure of tendons, ligaments, joint membranes and connective tissue.)

What foods is it found in?

- Gelatine
- Cheese
- Wheat
- Sunflower seeds
- Peanuts, almonds
- Oats

Useful information

Vitamins B3 and C are needed to enable the body to use proline. When the body is deficient in vitamin C, proline is lost in the urine. The body can synthesize ornithine from proline.

Colostrum, immunity and allergies

A proline-rich polypeptide, known as Colostrinin or PRP, first isolated from sheep colostrum, has been shown to restore balance in a number of immune functions in humans as well as animals. PRP contains 25% proline. Besides its effects on immunity, PRP also shows the ability to improve mental function and behavior in elderly rats, humans, and chickens. The authors conclude that it can be a valuable aid to the treatment of Alzheimer's disease[1]. In animal studies, PRP also decreased allergic responses to extracts from ragweed, pollen grains and house dust mites[2].

Eye disease

Five patients with gyrate atrophy of the choroid and retina of the eye were studied in order to investigate the possible therapeutic effects of vitamin B6 or proline supplements. There was no improvement in the one patient given B6 supplementation alone, or in another patient given both B6 and proline. Supplementary proline given alone minimized the progression of gyrate atrophy in the youngest patient and halted the progression in two others. The researchers conclude that supplementary proline may possibly lessen the progression of lesions in gyrate atrophy[3].

SUPPLEMENTS

How to use proline supplements

The main potential use for proline supplements is, along with arginine and glycine, in the healing of wounds and injuries and after surgery. Since gelatine is 19 per cent glycine, 12 per cent proline and 6 per cent arginine, it is an excellent natural supplement for wound-healing amino acids, although not suitable for vegetarians. It can be made into delicious desserts, or simply stirred into hot soups.

The usual recommended dose for pure proline supplements is 500-1500 mg per day.

How safe are proline supplements?

There are no known problems with proline supplements.

Proline content of common foods in grams per 100 g

Gelatine, dry	12.30
Cheese, cheddar	2.81
Wheat flour, whole-grain	1.42
Sunflower seeds, hulled	1.18
Peanuts, dry roasted	1.05
Almonds, raw	0.97
Oats	0.93
Beef, ground, extra-lean (approx. 21% fat)	0.90
Chicken meat, raw	0.88
Pork, composite of various cuts, trimmed, raw	0.81
Tuna, skipjack, fresh, raw	0.78
Brazil nuts, raw	0.76
Cornmeal, whole-grain, yellow	0.71
Walnuts, raw	0.71
Salmon, Atlantic, farmed, raw	0.70
Prawns, boiled	0.69
Herring, Atlantic, raw	0.64
Yoghurt, plain, low-fat	0.62
Eggs, hard-boiled	0.50
Buckwheat flour, whole groat	0.48
Tofu, raw, with calcium sulphate	0.44
Lentils, boiled	0.38
Chick peas, boiled	0.37
Mushrooms, raw	0.20
Beans, baked	0.20
Cabbage, boiled, drained	0.20
Broccoli, boiled, drained	0.12
Rice, brown, long-grain, boiled	0.12
Apricots, raw	0.10
Avocados, raw	0.08
Potatoes, peeled, boiled	0.06
Oranges, raw	0.05
Beetroot (beets) boiled, drained	0.04
Onions, boiled, drained	0.04
Bananas, raw	0.04
Peppers, sweet, green, raw	0.04
Aubergine (eggplant) boiled, drained	0.03
Carrots, boiled, drained	0.03
Apples, raw with skin	0.01

Source: USDA National Nutrient Database for Standard Reference, Release 28

Serine

What does the body use serine for?

- As a neurotransmitter
- To synthesize human protein
- To metabolize methionine
- To make phospholipids, sphingolipids, ethanolamine and choline
- Combines with carbohydrates to form glycoproteins
- Combines with homocysteine to form cystathione (with the help of vitamin B6)
- Can be metabolized to pyruvate and used to make energy
- Involved in DNA synthesis and provides a source of methyl groups for DNA.

In the form of phosphatidylserine, serine is highly concentrated in all cell membranes (the major work surfaces of cells). Phosphatidylserine (PS) is one of the five phospholipids, fatty substances which are important structural components of cell membranes and lipoproteins (proteins used to transport fats). Phospholipids hold the proteins and components of the cell membranes together and enable fat-soluble substances, including vitamins and hormones, to pass easily in and out of cells. Phosphatidylserine plays a key role in the electrical stability of cell membranes, especially brain cells, where it makes up about 70 per cent of nerve tissue. There it aids in the storage, release and activity of many vital neurotransmitters and their receptors. Phosphatidylserine has several unique functions, including:

- Upkeep and restoration of nerve cell membranes, which are involved in generating and transmitting electrical currents and in relaying the currents from cell to cell.
- Supporting the enzymes that regulate the balance between sodium and potassium and between calcium and magnesium.
- Activating the receptors on cell surfaces which enable the cell to respond to chemical messengers.
- Involvement in cell-to-cell communication and the regulation of nerve cell growth.
- Stimulates the release of dopamine
- Increases the production of acetylcholine (needed for learning and memory)
- Enhances brain glucose metabolism
- Reduces cortisol levels
- Boosts the activity of nerve growth factor (NGF).

Due to its key role in the membranes of the mitochondria—the part of the cell where energy is made, PS also plays a vital role in energy production[1].

Methionine is required for the formation of phospholipids from PS. Phospholipids containing choline are known as lecithins, while those containing ethanolamine or serine are known as cephalins.

What foods is it found in?

- Gelatine
- Cheese
- Peanuts
- Sunflower seeds
- Almonds
- Eggs
- Walnuts

Serine can also be made in the human body from glycine, with the aid of vitamin B3, B6 and folic acid.

Useful information

Over the adult life span, individuals can lose as much as 50 per cent of their ability to perform everyday tasks related to memory and thought. Because of PS's special role in the cell membranes of nerve cells, a number of clinical trials have been carried out, to see if PS can combat age-related declines in memory, learning and concentration[2,3,4]. Results are very encouraging, and the 'cognitive age' can be reduced by up to 12 years. In other words someone with the mental function of a 64 year-old can be restored to the mental function of a 52 year-old by taking PS supplements for 12 weeks[6]. Improvements are measured by assessing:

- Telephone number recall
- Misplaced objects recall
- Paragraph recall
- Ability to concentrate while reading, conversing, performing tasks.

PS appears to be able to boost the alpha rhythm of the brain by an average of 15-20 per cent[7]. This rhythm is often found to be lowered in ageing and decline of mental functions.

In rat studies, PS supplements have been shown to stimulate the release of acetylcholine and dopamine (major neurotransmitters required for memory function).

Alzheimer's disease

Research using PS supplementation shows that it can significantly improve several cognitive functions compared to placebo. Differences are more dramatic among patients with less severe impairment, suggesting that PS may be most useful in the early stages of Alzheimer's disease[8,9,10,11,12,13].

Stress and sleep

Research suggests that phosphatidylserine may have potential for the treatment of stress related disorders[14,15,16].

Cortisol is known as the stress hormone. Many researchers advocate the use of phosphatidylserine to lower cortisol. However, some have found that the phosphorylated form of serine has a much stronger cortisol-lowering impact and is one of a very few substances that can permanently subdue really stubborn cortisol elevation after only a few weeks or months of use. This makes it a valuable treatment for insomnia caused by high cortisol levels[17].

ADHD

Phosphatidylserine can significantly reduce ADHD symptoms in children, and can perform better than commonly prescribed ADHD drugs, improving attention, hyperactivity, impulsive behaviors and short-term auditory memory. Researchers believe that ADHD is linked with phospholipid and fatty acid deficiencies causing abnormal brain cell structure and abnormal function[18].

SUPPLEMENTS

How to use serine supplements

Serine supplements are taken in the form of phosphatidylserine. Most clinical trials have gained their results by using 100 mg PS, 3 times a day.

How safe are serine supplements?

In clinical trials using PS supplements, no significant side effects have been reported. In rare cases, taking 200 mg or more in one dose can cause nausea, due to the stimulation of dopamine release. This can be minimized by taking PS with meals.

Serine content of common foods in grams per 100 g

Gelatine, dry	2.61
Cheese, cheddar	1.46
Peanuts, dry roasted	1.17
Sunflower seeds, hulled	1.08
Almonds, raw	1.01
Eggs, hard-boiled	0.94
Walnuts, raw	0.93
Tuna, skipjack, fresh, raw	0.90
Prawns, boiled	0.82
Salmon, Atlantic, farmed, raw	0.81
Pork, composite of various cuts, trimmed, raw	0.78
Oats	0.75
Brazil nuts, raw	0.75
Chicken meat, raw	0.74
Herring, Atlantic, raw	0.73
Beef, ground, extra-lean (approx. 21% fat)	0.69
Buckwheat flour, whole groat	0.65
Wheat flour, whole-grain	0.65
Chick peas, boiled	0.45
Lentils, boiled	0.42
Cornmeal, whole-grain, yellow	0.39
Tofu, raw, with calcium sulphate	0.38
Yoghurt, plain, low-fat	0.33
Beans, baked	0.26
Rice, brown, long-grain, boiled	0.13
Mushrooms, raw	0.13
Broccoli, boiled, drained	0.11
Apricots, raw	0.08
Avocados, raw	0.08
Potatoes, peeled, boiled	0.08
Beetroot (beets) boiled, drained	0.06
Cabbage, boiled, drained	0.06
Bananas, raw	0.05
Onions, boiled, drained	0.04
Carrots, boiled, drained	0.04
Peppers, sweet, green, raw	0.04
Aubergine (eggplant) boiled, drained	0.03
Oranges, raw	0.03
Apples, raw with skin	0.01

Source: USDA National Nutrient Database for Standard Reference, Release 28

Taurine

What does the body use taurine for?

- Inhibitory neurotransmitter
- Stabilizes calcium in the brain and elsewhere
- Eye health
- Liver detoxification, especially for aldehydes and chlorine compounds
- Antioxidant
- Stabilizes cell membranes
- Facilitates the passage of sodium, potassium and calcium ions in and out of cells
- Combines with bile acids, keeping them soluble and allowing them to be excreted
- Helps to form bile salts
- Controls renin, thus helping to control blood pressure
- Controls levels of glutamic acid
- Promotes lactation in nursing mothers
- Stimulates the release of stomach acid
- Enhances sperm motility
- Enhances insulin activity

Taurine is one of the sulphur amino acids. Unlike the others it is not incorporated into muscle proteins but it is the second most abundant free amino acid in the brain. Within the brain taurine is concentrated in the taste and smell centre, the memory centre and the pineal gland. It is present in cell membranes, helping to stabilize them electrically.

This role may account for taurine's usefulness in the treatment of epilepsy, seizures and convulsions. After GABA, taurine is the second most important inhibitory neurotransmitter in the brain, helping to control the electrical impulses which pass along nerve cells. It is also found in large amounts in the eyes, and stabilizes the nerve cell membranes of the retina.

Taurine is the most abundant amino acid in the heart muscle. When taurine levels are low there, imbalances of sodium, potassium, calcium and magnesium occur and when glucose is introduced, potassium and sodium leave the cell and the sodium/calcium ratio inside the cell rises, causing abnormal heart rhythms. Taurine reverses the depletion of calcium and potassium.

In the liver taurine combines with bile acids (which are largely made from cholesterol) to form bile salts. These aid the digestion of fats in the small intestine.

One of taurine's most important roles is in liver detoxification. It helps to prevent the formation of toxic aldehydes and works as an antioxidant, especially for the hypochlorite free radical, which comes from chlorine.

What foods is it found in?

- Meat and organ meats
- Fish
- Cows' milk and human breast milk

Figures for the taurine content of foods are not yet available in standard amino acid reference works.

Except for young babies, the human body is able to make taurine from the amino acid cysteine (with the aid of vitamin B6) although it is not known whether this is always enough for our requirements. Infant formula feeds should always be enriched with taurine at least to the levels found in human breast milk. In the nursing mother, taurine increases blood levels of the hormone prolactin, which triggers the production and release of milk.

Domestic cats are not able to produce taurine in their bodies and must obtain it from their food. It is wise to ensure that cheap commercial pet foods which may contain only 5 per cent meat and are bulked out with gelatine provide adequate taurine.

Useful information

Factors which can encourage taurine deficiency include
- The food additive monosodium glutamate
- Lack of adequate zinc, vitamin A and vitamin B6
- Lack of methionine, or of nutrients needed for methionine metabolism
- Kidney problems, including inflammation of the kidney ducts, or damage due to over-acidity of the blood (acidosis) can result in excessive losses of taurine via the urine.
- Poor protein digestion or absorption
- Breast-feeding

A vitamin B6 deficiency, which is relatively common, results in high levels of the amino acid beta-alanine. This causes excessive losses of taurine through the urine.

Heart

Taurine supplementation is very popular in the far east. A number of studies show that it retards the initiation and progression of atherosclerosis[1].

Because of its role in heart function, taurine has been successfully used in supplement form to combat congestive heart failure. In a study published in the journal *Clinical Cardiology*, patients with congestive heart failure took either a placebo (a dummy pill) or 2,000 mg of taurine three times a day. The supplemented patients experienced significant improvements in their heart's ability to pump blood. None of them worsened during the taurine treatment, while 29 per cent of the placebo subjects did[2].

Taurine regulates calcium and potassium in heart muscle cells. This in turn regulates nerve impulses in the heart. Taurine also acts as a heart stimulant and encourages the excretion of sodium and water. Taurine has the ability to inhibit abnormal heart rhythms caused by excessive adrenaline and at the same time prevents adrenaline from depleting potassium in the heart muscle. It has been described as a natural calcium channel blocker (a type of drug used to treat high blood pressure and angina).

Brain

It used to be believed that the body could not produce new brain cells—that we will never have more than those we are born with, and that these will slowly deteriorate and decline as we age.

Researchers are now showing that this is not true. Recent research reveals that taurine can promote new brain cell formation. In animal studies taurine supplements have been used to trigger new brain cells to grow in the hippocampus, the area of the brain most concerned with memory. Taurine increased the growth of brain cells (neurons) by activating 'sleeping' stem cells. It may also be able to increase the survival of neurons[3-8].

As well as promoting the growth of new brain cells, taurine protects neurites—tiny projections that help neurons communicate with each other. Neurites maximize connections along which electrical impulses flow to support memory, feeling and thinking. Over time, chemical stressors and toxins can damage these neurites[9]. A lab study suggests that taurine may be able to restore normal neurite growth in neurons which have been exposed to toxic chemicals[10].

Taurine supplementation has been found to help combat epileptic seizures. It is not known how it exerts this effect. Possible explanations are that taurine may help by balancing the excitatory amino acid glutamic acid and the inhibitory amino acid GABA. Or by stabilizing the minerals which govern electrical activity within the nervous system.

In one research study, taurine supplementation was found to reduce dementia in elderly people[11]. In another small study, 15 out of 16 alcoholics given taurine supplements to aid alcohol withdrawal became rapidly free of delerium tremens, hallucinations and seizures[12].

Research is beginning to emerge suggesting that low taurine levels (exacerbated by L-dopa treatment) may be involved in the development or progress of Parkinson's disease[13].

Hearing

Taurine plays a vital role in hearing. Much hearing damage occurs in the hair-like nerve cells that convert sound waves into the electrical energy that is perceived in our brain. Like other nerve cells, these depend on the flow of calcium ions into and out of the cell. Taurine helps restore and control this calcium ion flow[14,15].

Taurine may be able to eliminate ringing in the ears caused by tinnitus[16].

Eyes

Dr Merril J Allen, Professor Emeritus of Indiana University School of Optometry in Illinois, uses taurine supplements together with bilberry extract and stimulation with micro-electrical currents to treat and reverse the disease process in retinitis pigmentosa[17].

Gallstones

Another important use for taurine supplements is to reduce cholesterol levels by assisting the body with cholesterol excretion via bile. Taurine helps to keep bile soluble and thus may help to prevent gallstones from forming. Those with gallbladder disease may need supplemental taurine to help dissolve gallstones which have already formed.

Liver detoxification

Taurine-deficient individuals may become very sensitive to aldehydes, chlorine, bleach and other similar chemicals, because taurine is needed to help process these substances and the hypochlorite free radicals they produce[18]. It combines with toxins in a process called acylation, and aids their excretion. Animal studies suggest that taking taurine before drinking alcohol can help to prevent the formation of toxic acetaldehyde[19].

Metabolic syndrome and diabetes

Obese people can have up to 41 per cent and diabetic people up to 40 per cent lower taurine levels compared with healthy individuals[20,21].

Taurine supplementation is an effective treatment for many of the abnormalities involved in the prediabetic condition known as metabolic syndrome. It is also being increasingly considered as a useful tool for both the prevention and treatment of diabetes and its complications[22].

Kidneys

Taurine seems to have a protective effect for the kidneys, against both toxic damage, and damage caused by diabetes[23].

Cystic fibrosis

Cystic fibrosis is a disease in which the respiratory system and the pancreas produce large amounts of thick mucus, resulting in chronic chest infections and poor digestion. In a study administering taurine supplements to cystic fibrosis patients, weight and height increased in 50 per cent of the patients, and fat malabsorption improved[24].

SUPPLEMENTS

How to use taurine supplements

1000 mg per day is probably adequate for most purposes. A good combination product for those taking taurine for a heart condition is magnesium taurate, since magnesium can also help to stabilize the heart's electrical activity.

If taurine supplements are not available, n-acetyl cysteine (NAC) supplements will raise taurine levels, since one of the main factions of NAC in the body is to convert into taurine.

To aid absorption, taurine supplements are best not taken at the same time as protein or with other amino acid supplements, especially glutamic acid or aspartic acid.

How safe are taurine supplements?

Based on the available published human clinical trial data, the evidence for the absence of adverse effects is strong for taurine at supplemental intakes up to 3 grams per day[25].

Temporary itching has been reported by psoriasis patients taking 2 grams of taurine daily, and some epileptic patients have reported nausea, headache, dizziness, and gait disturbances at dosages of 1.5 grams daily. Taurine supplements should not be taken with aspirin, as they can increase stomach acidity. Taurine supplementation may reduce the painkilling effects of morphine, perhaps by hastening the clearance of morphine from the body. This could perhaps make it useful in helping to speed up the withdrawal process when treating morphine addiction.

Threonine

What does the body use threonine for?

- Making serine and glycine
- Can be turned into glucose if needed for energy
- Required for transport of copper to the body's cells
- Linking with carbohydrates to form glycoprotein

Threonine is one of the five amino acids that link with carbohydrates to form glycoproteins. Glycoproteins are required for proper immune system function. Some research has indicated that threonine may be especially important for the thymus gland.

What foods is it found in?

- Gelatine
- Meat, fish
- Cheese
- Sunflower seeds
- Peanuts
- Almonds

The human body cannot make threonine and must obtain it from the diet.

Useful information

Threonine is a very slowly absorbed amino acid and can be particularly deficient in individuals with intestinal malabsorption. In experimental animals a severe threonine deficiency causes neurological (nerve function) symptoms such as difficulty in walking.

The Brain Bio Center in New Jersey reports that of fifteen patients found to have low threonine levels, all fifteen were suffering from severe clinical depression. Several of these patients responded to threonine supplementation[1].

Spasticity

Threonine supplementation (500 mg per day) was given for 12 months to six patients suffering from genetic spasticity. This was followed by a 4-month observation period without medication. All six patients showed partial improvement of spasticity, knee jerks and muscle spasms. The range of overall improvement, objectively measured, was 7-30% for upper limbs, and 25-67% for lower limbs. No toxic clinical or biochemical side effects were encountered. Threonine, a precursor of glycine, produced the same effect on spasticity as that previously observed with glycine. The authors conclude that threonine deserves a controlled trial in genetic cases of spasticity[2].

In studies on patients suffering from spasticity as a result of multiple sclerosis or spinal cord injury, L-threonine supplementation also had an antispastic effect at a dosage of three grams per day. This is thought to be due to threonine's ability to enhance glycine-related inhibition of nerve impulses[3,4].

Brain function

In recent years, scientists are discovering the importance of the mineral magnesium for brain functions such as learning and memory. Magnesium deficiency is widespread[5] and although this mineral can be supplemented, magnesium supplements are not very efficiently absorbed into the brain and nervous system. A new form of magnesium supplement where magnesium is bonded with the amino acid threonine, appears to get round this problem. Compared with magnesium citrate supplements (previously considered the most highly absorbable form) magnesium-L-threonate supplementation in trials on elderly animals brought improvements of 15 per cent for short-term memory, and 54 per cent for long-term memory. In young animals the figures rose to 18 per cent for short-term and 100 per cent for long-term memory[6].

SUPPLEMENTS

How to use threonine supplements

L-threonine supplements are not generally available, as pllenty of threonine can be obtained from food sources.

The manufacturers of magnesium-L-threonate sell this product in capsules, each providing 144 mg magnesium. Two of these a day should be adequate for most individuals. Please note that the tolerable upper limit for magnesium supplementation is 350 mg per day, so it is not advisable to exceed this dose.

Supplemental magnesium can also interfere with the action of certain medications, so please consult your doctor before taking them.

Threonine content of common foods in grams per 100 g

Gelatine, dry	1.40
Tuna, skipjack, fresh, raw	0.96
Sunflower seeds, hulled	0.93
Chicken meat, raw	0.90
Cheese, cheddar	0.89
Salmon, Atlantic, farmed, raw	0.87
Pork, composite of various cuts, trimmed, raw	0.86
Prawns, boiled	0.85
Peanuts, dry roasted	0.81
Herring, Atlantic, raw	0.79
Beef, ground, extra-lean (approx. 21% fat)	0.74
Almonds, raw	0.68
Walnuts, raw	0.60
Eggs, hard-boiled	0.60
Oats	0.58
Buckwheat flour, whole groat	0.48
Brazil nuts, raw	0.46
Wheat flour, whole-grain	0.40
Tofu, raw, with calcium sulphate	0.33
Chick peas, boiled	0.33
Lentils, boiled	0.32
Cornmeal, whole-grain, yellow	0.31
Yoghurt, plain, low-fat	0.22
Beans, baked	0.20
Mushrooms, raw	0.13
Broccoli, boiled, drained	0.10
Rice, brown, long-grain, boiled	0.10
Avocados, raw	0.07
Potatoes, peeled, boiled	0.06
Beetroot (beets) boiled, drained	0.05
Apricots, raw	0.05
Carrots, boiled, drained	0.04
Cabbage, boiled, drained	0.04
Bananas, raw	0.03
Onions, boiled, drained	0.03
Peppers, sweet, green, raw	0.03
Aubergine (eggplant) boiled, drained	0.03
Oranges, raw	0.02
Apples, raw with skin	0.01

Source: USDA National Nutrient Database for Standard Reference, Release 28

L-Tryptophan, L-5-Hydroxytryptophan (5-HTP) and Melatonin

What does the body use tryptophan for?

- Making the neurotransmitter serotonin
- Making the neurotransmitter, neuro-hormone and antioxidant melatonin
- Making vitamin B3
- Making picolinic acid, which aids zinc absorption

Tryptophan cannot be made by the human body and must be obtained from the diet. It is best known for its role in the production of 5-hydroxytryptamine or serotonin, a brain neurotransmitter involved in sleep promotion and sometimes known as the 'happiness hormone'. Serotonin is made with the aid of vitamin B6, magnesium and a form of folic acid known as biopterin. It is known as the happiness hormone because SSRI-type antidepressant drugs work by maintaining high levels of serotonin in the body.

Once dietary tryptophan is converted in the body to serotonin it can be made into melatonin by two enzymes in the pineal gland. Melatonin aids sleep, and its production is stimulated by a lack of light. Bright light can decrease its production. Melatonin also has powerful antioxidant properties.

Approximately 1.5 to 2 per cent of absorbed tryptophan can also be converted to vitamin B3 within the body, with the aid of vitamin B6, C, glutamine, iron and magnesium.

In the pancreas, a small amount of the body's tryptophan becomes picolinic acid, which assists with zinc absorption and transport. People with a deficiency of vitamin B6 or tryptophan cannot absorb zinc.

What foods is it found in?

- Sunflower seeds
- Cheese
- Meat, fish
- Oats
- Brazil nuts and peanuts

Serotonin

Serotonin levels decline as we age[1]. This may be because levels of inflammatory cytokines increase with age. These cytokines activate an enzyme which breaks down tryptophan. The effects of this enzyme can be reduced by ensuring that we get an adequate intake of vitamin B3[2].

The concentration of serotonin in the brain is directly proportional to the concentration of tryptophan. Subnormal levels of serotonin due either to tryptophan deficiency or to poor metabolism of tryptophan can cause:

- Disordered sleep patterns
- Insomnia
- Anxiety or depression
- Abnormal appetite and food craving
- Hypersensitivity to light, sound and other external stimuli
- Excessive sensitivity to pain
- Attention deficits and behaviour disorders

If tryptophan is not properly absorbed from the intestines, due to intestinal problems such as chronic inflammation or coeliac disease (gluten allergy), bacteria can act on the tryptophan, producing indican. Levels of indican can be measured in the urine as a test for tryptophan malabsorption. In severe malabsorption, gut bacteria can also produce from tryptophan substances called methyl tryptamines, which cause hallucinations and other symptoms of mental illness. People with coeliac disease, who suffer from severe diarrhoea due to gluten allergy or sometimes due to carbohydrate intolerance, are prone to experience such mental symptoms.

The consumption of carbohydrates (e.g. sugar) with protein encourages the uptake of tryptophan into the brain. This is because carbohydrate leads to insulin release. Insulin lowers the blood levels of tyrosine and other amino acids which compete with tryptophan for entry into the brain. Larger amounts of tryptophan can then pass through the blood brain barrier. Because tryptophan is converted into serotonin in the brain, a 'sugar high' may be experienced after a meal, drink or snack which causes a rapid rise in insulin, and this may pave the way to sugar addiction.

It is important for people with chronic fatigue syndrome to avoid 'sugar highs', to avoid consuming excess tryptophan and especially to avoid consuming carbohydrate at the same time as protein. This dietary strategy may help to control the excessive drowsiness which is often associated with chronic fatigue syndrome, by keeping down serotonin levels in the brain[3].

Autism

Serotonin promotes normal social behavior and helps individuals to accurately assess emotional social cues—abilities that are lacking in autism. High tryptophan and serotonin levels are often found in autistic children. But the higher the levels, the worse tends to be their psychiatric rating. Autistic children appear to have some defect in tryptophan-serotonin metabolism in the brain, which may account for some of their clinical and behavioural abnormalities[4]. This abnormality may be related to a vitamin D deficiency. Researchers have discovered that vitamin D3 is needed to activate a gene that converts tryptophan to serotonin in the brain. Vitamin D also controls enzymes which reduce the production of serotonin. A vitamin D deficiency could explain why people with autism often have high levels of serotonin in the blood but low levels in the brain. According to a 2006 NHANES report, 96% of Americans not taking vitamin and mineral supplements have insufficient vitamin D levels[5].

Mental illness

The Brain Bio Center in New Jersey, USA, has for decades specialized in the treatment of mental disorders by adjusting body biochemistry. It was one of the pioneers of the view that some individuals with clinical depression or schizophrenia have a poor balance between the neurotransmitters dopamine (derived from tyrosine) and serotonin (derived from tryptophan). Suicidal patients and those with agitated depression often show low serotonin levels. When dopamine is in excess and serotonin levels are low, tryptophan supplementation produces clinical improvements, presumably by balancing the excess dopamine[2]. Tryptophan and 5-HTP are frequently used as antidepressants and have been shown to elevate brain serotonin levels and enhance both mood and a sense of well-being[6].

Theoretically, the combination of tryptophan with tyrosine could have potential for even more marked energy and mood-elevating effects[7]. Orthomolecular psychiatrists (those who use nutrients in preference to drugs) say that prescribing 1 gram of L-tyrosine in the morning and 1 gram of L-tryptophan in the evening can probably mimic the effects of most pharmaceutical antidepressants[8]. Most of these pharmaceuticals work by manipulating levels of dopamine and its related compounds.

For those with depression caused by seasonal affective disorder, tryptophan can produce benefits equal to those of light therapy[9].

Tryptophan in the form of 5-HTP has been shown in a randomized double blind study to be as effective as the drug fluoxetine for clinical depression, though it takes two weeks to start working[10].

Schizophrenics with a dopamine excess and low histamine levels may respond to tryptophan, according to the Brain Bio Center. In these cases tryptophan probably works by balancing dopamine excess[8].

Mania too can respond to tryptophan therapy. Lithium, which is a drug normally prescribed for mania, helps the transmission of nerve impulses which depend on serotonin. Patients tell the Brain Bio Center that combining night-time lithium with 1-3 grams of tryptophan enhances the benefit of the lithium[8]. Dr Chouinard from McGill University is of the opinion that tryptophan used alone is as effective as lithium[11]. Aggression (see below) and anxiety[12] can also result from low tryptophan levels.

Aggression

This is one of the most intensively-studied topics in tryptophan research. Studies are consistently finding that low tryptophan levels can aggravate a tendency to aggressive, hostile behaviour, and tryptophan supplementation can reduce it. In one research study, people with a high aggression score were given two amino acid drinks; one designed to raise tryptophan levels, and the other to deplete them. On assessment it was found that the subjects became more hostile, aggressive and quarrelsome after tryptophan depletion, and less so after tryptophan supplementation. In another study, aggressive psychiatric patients treated with up to six grams per day of L-tryptophan showed a significant reduction in the need for antipsychotic and sedative injections[13,14].

Young people with ADHD may show inappropriate aggression in response to very little provocation. Tryptophan depletion can aggravate this problem[15].

Tryptophan depletion also enhances self-injurious behaviour[16].

Supplementation with 3 grams/day of tryptophan has been found to reduce quarrelsome behaviour and enhance socially constructive behaviours[17].

Aggression experienced by women as a premenstrual problem can also be aggravated by tryptophan depletion[18].

Since depleting tryptophan does not appear to induce aggression in those who are not easily provoked into aggressive behaviour, it is thought that the primary effects of the depletion are related to increased impulsiveness[13]. Rapid lowering of tryptophan by administering a mixture of essential amino acids excluding tryptophan, does appear to increase impulsiveness and to decrease discriminating ability in normal individuals[19].

Effects of alcohol

Alcohol-induced memory impairment can be reduced by consuming a tryptophan supplement before the alcohol. This suggests that this impairment may be due to a reduction in brain serotonin, caused by alcohol[20]. Aggression after alcohol consumption may also be explained by serotonin depletion[21].

In a study involving recovering alcoholic patients, it was found that the patients had severely depleted L-tryptophan levels accompanied by clinical depression. Tryptophan supplements considerably alleviated this depression[22].

Parkinson's disease

Some researchers have used tryptophan supplements to treat Parkinson's disease for two reasons:
- The deficiency of serotonin-dependent nerve impulses which occurs in these patients
- The side-effects of the antiparkinsonian drugs

Some dramatic improvements have been reported[23]. Doses of 150 mg to 1.5 grams per day have been shown to reduce the psychotic behaviour associated with the anti-parkinsonian drug L-dopa. Tryptophan dosages of four grams a day can also reduce or prevent the feeling of inner restlessness and need to move[24].

Melatonin supplements may help to preserve cells' ability to make dopamine and to reduce the accumulation of the destructive proteins found in Parkinson's disease[25,26].

Multiple sclerosis

MS patients often report that mental stress exacerbates their symptoms and even provokes attacks of their disease. Aggravation of the symptoms does not always occur during the stress, but may occur on the rebound. Stress causes increased cortisol production by the adrenal glands and increased metabolism of serotonin in the brain. In chronic MS, levels of available tryptophan in the blood plasma and cerebrospinal fluid are reduced and may be reduced even further in those who are stressed. Since the reason for this lack of tryptophan availability is not known, tryptophan supplementation may be of value to help reduce the effects of stress on the disease by improving serotonin levels[27].

Pain

The nucleus raphus magnus is a part of the brain responsible for inhibiting pain. It depends on serotonin and therefore tryptophan for optimal functioning. Although research studies have variable results, There is now growing evidence that tryptophan supplementation can enhance the action of the body's natural painkillers, the enkephalins and endorphins, to decrease the perception of pain and raise the body's pain tolerance thresholds[28].

Exercise tolerance

Strenuous physical exercise is associated with discomfort and pain. The tolerance for this pain is also regulated by the body's enkephalins and endorphins. Because serotonin affects the perception of pain through its effects on this system, the effects of supplementation with L-tryptophan on endurance and sensation of effort were investigated in a research study. Twelve healthy sportsmen were subjected to a work load corresponding to 80 per cent of their maximal oxygen uptake after receiving a placebo (inert substance) and after receiving an L-tryptophan supplement. The subjects ran on a treadmill until they were exhausted. The total exercise time, amount of exertion felt, maximum heart rate, peak oxygen consumption, pulse recovery rate, and post-exercise oxygen consumption were then assessed. The total exercise time was 49.4% greater after receiving L-tryptophan than after receiving the placebo. The subjects felt they had exerted themselves less while on tryptophan[29].

The researchers believed that these results could be due to an increased tolerance to pain as a result of L-tryptophan ingestion, but subsequent research on sports performance has shown that the effects of serotonin on the function of motor neurons may be a better explanation[30].

Weight problems

It is now known that low tryptophan levels result in food cravings, especially for carbohydrates. According to recent research, tryptophan supplementation has the opposite effect. 20 obese patients were randomly assigned to receive either 5-hydroxytryptophan (5-HTP) at a dosage of 900 mg a day, or a placebo (inert substance). (L-tryptophan is converted into 5-HTP before being made into serotonin.)

The study was double-blind, which meant that neither the test subjects nor the researchers knew which people had been given the tryptophan. It was carried out for two consecutive six-week periods. No diet was prescribed during the first period, but a calorie-controlled diet was recommended for the second.

Significant weight loss occurred in the tryptophan-supplemented group during both periods. Both their appetite and their carbohydrate intake were reduced. They felt satisfied by eating smaller amounts of food. The researchers, who were based at the Department of Internal Medicine at the University of Rome, concluded that these findings, together with the lack of side effects, suggest that 5-HTP may be safely used to treat obesity[31].

Tryptophan supplements can also decrease cravings and binge eating—especially for carbohydrates[32,33].

Other benefits

Supplementation of 5-HTP can improve sleep, fatigue, mood, and tender point counts in patients with fibromyalgia[34].

The SSRI drug Prozac, which works by maintaining high levels of serotonin in the body, is now a standard treatment for premenstrual syndrome (PMS). Tryptophan supplements may be a viable alternative[35].

Oestrogen increases the conversion of tryptophan to vitamin B3, which puts contraceptive pill users at risk of tryptophan deficiency. It has been estimated that in order to prevent this deficiency, contraceptive pill users need to consume at least 20 mg vitamin B6 per day (10 times the RDA). Tryptophan metabolism is highly dependent on vitamin B6[36].

Tryptophan is an effective treatment for insomnia[37,38]. Although tryptophan has sedative properties, it may not impair performance[39].

For resistant insomnia, and for agitated depression and schizophrenia, melatonin supplements (not available in the UK) may work better than tryptophan. Melatonin is often referred to as the 'anti-jet lag' supplement because it can help to reset the body clock when changing time zones.

SUPPLEMENTS

How to use tryptophan supplements

To aid sleep, take 500-1,000 mg 30 minutes before bed-time, with a little fruit juice to aid absorption into the brain. (Or melatonin 1-5 mg, half an hour to two hours before bed-time.) Take with 10 mg zinc, since enzymes that metabolize and store melatonin in the pineal gland are zinc-dependent.

For most other purposes, 500 mg taken twice a day is a typical dose. To aid absorption into the brain tryptophan should not be consumed at the same time as protein or with other amino acid supplements.

As a weight loss aid, take tryptophan supplements with fruit juice half an hour before meals.

Typical dosages of 5-HTP are 50 to 300 mg.

How safe are tryptophan supplements?

In 1990 L-tryptophan supplements were withdrawn from general sale for several years after supplies which were produced using genetically engineered bacteria led to cases of a disease known as eosinophilia myalgia syndrome. This process is no longer used to make tryptophan supplements.

Up to 4 grams a day of L-tryptophan rarely causes problems for adults. But do not take L-tryptophan without medical advice if you are taking anti-depressant drugs known as selective serotonin reuptake inhibitors (SSRIs). This combination could lead to serious side effects.

One study on monkeys found that while L-tryptophan supplementation reduced aggression, 5-HTP supplements increased it[40]. Tryptophan supplements also reduce the effects of morphine.

Excessive doses of 5-HTP supplementation may cause nausea and diarrhoea. In case of interaction, 5-HTP should not be taken at the same time as pharmaceutical medications. It is also best avoided by pregnant women. According to studies on rats, tryptophan supplementation can be toxic in individuals with adrenal insufficiency (poorly functioning adrenal glands).

Tryptophan content of common foods in grams per 100 g

Sunflower seeds, hulled	0.35
Cheese, cheddar	0.32
Prawns, boiled	0.29
Brazil nuts, raw	0.26
Chicken meat, raw	0.25
Tuna, skipjack, fresh, raw	0.25
Oats	0.23
Pork, composite of various cuts, trimmed, raw	0.23
Peanuts, dry roasted	0.23
Salmon, Atlantic, farmed, raw	0.22
Beef, ground, extra-lean (approx. 21% fat)	0.22
Wheat flour, whole-grain	0.21
Herring, Atlantic, raw	0.20
Almonds, raw	0.19
Buckwheat flour, whole groat	0.18
Walnuts, raw	0.17
Eggs, hard-boiled	0.15
Tofu, raw, with calcium sulphate	0.13
Chick peas, boiled	0.09
Lentils, boiled	0.08
Mushrooms, raw	0.07
Beans, baked	0.06
Cornmeal, whole-grain, yellow	0.06
Rice, brown, long-grain, boiled	0.03
Broccoli, boiled, drained	0.03
Yoghurt, plain, low-fat	0.03
Potatoes, peeled, boiled	0.03
Avocados, raw	0.02
Beetroot (beets) boiled, drained	0.02
Onions, boiled, drained	0.02
Apricots, raw	0.02
Bananas, raw	0.01
Carrots, boiled, drained	0.01
Peppers, sweet, green, raw	0.01
Cabbage, boiled, drained	0.01
Oranges, raw	0.01
Aubergine (eggplant) boiled, drained	0.01
Apples, raw with skin	0.00
Gelatine, dry	0.00

Source: USDA National Nutrient Database for Standard Reference, Release 28

L-Tyrosine

What does the body use L-tyrosine for?

- Making the hormones thyroxine, adrenaline, noradrenaline and dopamine, which is also a neurotransmitter
- Making enkephalins (the body's natural pain relievers)
- Making amino sugars

Tyrosine is made in the body from the amino acid phenylalanine and is the raw material of the three catecholamine hormones: adrenaline (epinephrine in the U.S.), noradrenaline (norepinephrine) and dopamine. These are involved in blood pressure control, alertness, mood, concentration and coping with stress.

Tyrosine is also used to make thyroid hormone, which is needed for growth and energy metabolism.

Tyrosine is broken down by the enzyme tyrosinase to yield melanin—the 'sun tan' pigment which protects against the harmful effects of sunlight. It is also the pigment in human hair.

Another enzyme known as tyrosine hydroxylase helps turn L-tyrosine to L-DOPA with the help of folic acid and iron. The activity of this enzyme can be as low as 10 per cent in people with Parkinson's disease, suggesting that one of more of the elements needed for the formation of L-DOPA are in insufficient quantities. Another enzyme converts L-DOPA to dopamine with the help of vitamin

B6. The activity of this enzyme rises and falls according to how much vitamin B6 is available.

What foods is it found in?

- Cheese
- Peanuts
- Fish, meat
- Sunflower seeds, almonds
- Oats
- Eggs

The artificial sweetener aspartame, which is found in many diet products, can lead to increased tyrosine levels in the brain. It contains the amino acid phenylalanine, which can be converted to tyrosine.

The use of oral contraceptives decreases tyrosine availability to the brain, which may lead to disturbances of mood, coping mechanisms, and appetite due to lower levels of noradrenaline (norepinephrine)[1].

Hormone deficiencies

A lack of catecholamine hormones can lead to low blood pressure, 'stress exhaustion', reduced sex drive and mental symptoms of apathy and depression. A deficiency of thyroid hormone leads to fatigue, weight gain and low body temperature. When these symptoms occur as a result of hormone deficiencies, they may respond to supplementation with tyrosine since it is the main raw material from which these hormones are derived. Many antidepressant drugs work by preventing the breakdown of hormones made from tyrosine.

Parkinson's disease

People with Parkinson's disease show a loss of the neurons which secrete dopamine, in the substantia nigra part of the brain. Symptoms are due to dopamine deficiency, and are usually not present until 80 per cent of these neurons are lost. Because tyrosine is the raw material for dopamine, some researchers have combined tyrosine supplements with conventional medications in patients with Parkinson's disease, and claim to obtain better clinical results with fewer side effects than with conventional treatments alone[2].

Raised homocysteine levels are a sign of B vitamin deficiencies. They are frequently found in Parkinson's disease, and can be raised even further by L-DOPA treatment, potentially worsening the condition. For this reason, B complex supplements are often recommended for those taking the drug[3].

Vitamin B6 is particularly important, as it is a co-factor for the enzyme which helps to form dopamine. Vitamin B6 supplements can improve several criteria in Parkinson's disease[4].

However if a patient is being treated with L-DOPA alone without the additional drug carbidopa, vitamin B6 supplements may cause L-DOPA to convert to dopamine too early, before it can cross the blood-brain barrier. This is undesirable, so it is best to take the supplements at a time of day furthest from the last dose of L-DOPA and to have periodic blood tests to make sure that excess dopamine is not accumulating in the bloodstream. The most effective form of vitamin B6 is pyridoxal-5' phosphate[5].

Vitamin D deficiency is also common in people with Parkinson's disease[6]. Recent animal studies have shown that the presence of a vitamin D deficiency while the brain is developing can affect the ability of dopamine-producing neurons to mature. Fortunately vitamin D supplementation can help to improve the production of tyrosine hydroxylase—the enzyme needed for dopamine synthesis. There is also consistent evidence that vitamin D aids the survival of dopamine-producing neurons which have been exposed to toxins[7]. Toxins such as carbon monoxide, herbicides, methanol, and insecticides are strongly linked to the development of Parkinson's disease.

L-theanine, is an amino acid found in green tea that can cross the blood-brain barrier and prevent damage to dopamine-producing cells. Green tea extracts can also inhibit enzymes which break down dopamine, thus reducing the severity of symptoms[8]. Not just Parkinson's disease but also other neurodegenerative diseases can benefit from the protection provided by green tea[9,10].

Addiction and stress

Dopamine (made from tyrosine) has been called the 'anti-stress molecule' and/or the 'pleasure molecule'. When released into the brain it stimulates a number of receptors, and this reduces feelings of stress and increases feelings of well-being.

Addictive behaviour has been linked to a dysfunction of dopamine. Known as the 'Reward Deficiency Syndrome', this dysfunction causes a lack of usual feelings of satisfaction, resulting in behaviours which increase brain dopamine levels, including overeating, heavy cigarette smoking, drug and alcohol abuse, gambling, and hyperactivity. Although there is a lack of research into the potential use of tyrosine supplementation to combat addiction, there has been great interest in investigating its effects against stress.

Research is currently in progress by the US military and aerospace authorities, using tyrosine supplements to counteract the stress and fatigue seen in sustained operations consisting of continuous work periods exceeding 12 hours and often involving sleep loss[11,12,13].

Heat, cold, sleep deprivation and noise can be major causes of stress. Tyrosine supplementation has been found to increase the ability to exercise in the heat[14]. It can also lessen the drop in brain performance caused by exposure to cold[15], and mitigate the effects of noise stress on mental function[16].

Mental function

The effects of the amino acid tyrosine on the performance of mental tasks were studied on a group of 21 cadets during a demanding military combat training course. Ten individuals received five daily doses of a protein-rich drink containing 2 grams of tyrosine, and 11 individuals received a carbohydrate rich drink with the same amount of calories. Assessments were made both immediately prior to the combat course and on the 6th day of the course. The group supplied with the tyrosine-rich drink performed better on a memory and a tracking task than the group supplied with the carbohydrate-rich drink. In addition, tyrosine decreased the systolic blood pressure. The researchers conclude that tyrosine supplements can reduce the effects of stress and fatigue on the performance of mental tasks[17] .

By increasing dopamine in the brain, tyrosine supplementation can also aid mental flexibility[18].

Tyrosine supplements can improve our ability to multitask[19].

Narcolepsy

In the experience of the Brain Bio Center in New Jersey, 100 per cent of people suffering from narcolepsy (who are continually falling asleep) benefit from tyrosine supplementation. Those with mild narcolepsy may improve by 50 to 75 per cent, while those with severe narcolepsy may improve by only 10 to 25 per cent and require additional medication[20]. The Brain Bio Center also reports that tyrosine is very helpful for restless leg syndrome, and for people who are trying to give up smoking.

Schizophrenia

According to the Brain Bio Center, high levels of copper in the body can lead to an increased turnover of tyrosine to dopamine, plus a pronounced reduction in histamine levels and possibly a tyrosine shortage. They report that a combination of high dopamine, low histamine and high copper is common in people with schizophrenia. They treat it by supplementation with zinc (which competes with copper) and with branched-chain amino acids, which compete with tyrosine for entry into the brain[20].

Depression

Trials using tyrosine supplementation against clinical depression have shown encouraging results. In a 1988 research study, 12 patients with dopamine-deficiency depression treated with tyrosine showed a return to normal mood on the first day of treatment[21,22]. Another researcher reports that two women with long-standing clinical depression which had failed to respond to most conventional treatments—with the exception of amphetamines—were able to discontinue (in one case) or virtually discontinue (in the other case) their amphetamines within two weeks of starting L-tyrosine at a dosage of 100 mg per kilo of body weight once a day before breakfast[23].

Use of the contraceptive pill is known to deplete tyrosine levels, which may lead to depression. It is thought that oestrogen may increase levels of the enzyme tyrosine aminotransferase, which enhances the breakdown of tyrosine in the liver[24].

Thyroid

High tyrosine levels can also be present in people suffering from hyperthyroidism—an excess of thyroid hormone, which is one of the hormones derived from tyrosine. Conversely, people suffering from the opposite condition, hypothyroidism, may have low tyrosine levels.

SUPPLEMENTS

How to use L-tyrosine supplements

For most purposes a dose of 1 gram am and pm should suffice. Tyrosine supplements are best taken away from food and separately from other amino acid supplements (especially tryptophan, carnitine and the branched-chain amino acids) to avoid competition for entry into the brain. The body's ability to use tyrosine depends on the presence of adequate vitamin C, copper and a form of folic acid known as biopterin, so care should be taken that these nutrients are not in short supply. Elevated tyrosine levels in the blood may be a sign of a vitamin C or folic acid deficiency.

How safe are L-tyrosine supplements?

In military research, tyrosine doses of up to 150 mg per kilo of body weight (the equivalent of 90 grams of tyrosine for a small adult) have been given orally to humans without any side effects.

Tyrosine supplements should not be taken by people on MAO inhibitor drugs (which inhibit the breakdown of hormones made from tyrosine) or those suffering from malignant melanoma, a type of cancer associated with high levels of melanin. The Brain Bio Center also recommends the avoidance of tyrosine by individuals suffering from schizophrenia because they may already have high dopamine levels.

Tyrosine content of common foods in grams per 100 g

Cheese, cheddar	1.20
Peanuts, dry roasted	0.96
Tuna, skipjack, fresh, raw	0.74
Chicken meat, raw	0.72
Prawns, boiled	0.70
Salmon, Atlantic, farmed, raw	0.67
Sunflower seeds, hulled	0.67
Pork, composite of various cuts, trimmed, raw	0.65
Herring, Atlantic, raw	0.61
Oats	0.57
Beef, ground, extra-lean (approx. 21% fat)	0.55
Almonds, raw	0.53
Eggs, hard-boiled	0.51
Brazil nuts, raw	0.46
Walnuts, raw	0.41
Wheat flour, whole-grain	0.40
Cornmeal, whole-grain, yellow	0.33
Gelatine, dry	0.30
Tofu, raw, with calcium sulphate	0.27
Yoghurt, plain, low-fat	0.27
Lentils, boiled	0.24
Buckwheat flour, whole groat	0.23
Chick peas, boiled	0.22
Beans, baked	0.14
Rice, brown, long-grain, boiled	0.10
Broccoli, boiled, drained	0.07
Potatoes, peeled, boiled	0.06
Mushrooms, raw	0.06
Avocados, raw	0.05
Beetroot (beets) boiled, drained	0.04
Onions, boiled, drained	0.03
Apricots, raw	0.03
Bananas, raw	0.02
Aubergine (eggplant) boiled, drained	0.02
Carrots, boiled, drained	0.02
Peppers, sweet, green, raw	0.02
Cabbage, boiled, drained	0.02
Oranges, raw	0.02
Apples, raw with skin	0.00

Source: USDA National Nutrient Database for Standard Reference, Release 28

Valine

What does the body use valine for?

- With other branched-chain amino acids, valine is a major component of collagen
- Maintains and stimulates the synthesis of body muscle and other types of protein
- Prevents the breakdown of body proteins in trauma states

Valine is one of the three branched-chain amino acids. The other two are leucine and isoleucine. It cannot be made by the human body, and must be consumed through food. The BCAAs decrease the rate of breakdown and utilization of other amino acids and help to prevent hypercatabolism— the breaking down of the body's tissues which can occur after major trauma. The BCAAs are particularly needed by the muscles, and to cope with major stresses such as surgery and severe injuries and infections. If needed for energy, valine can be broken down into glucose.

What foods is it found in?

- Gelatine
- Cheese
- Sunflower seeds
- Meat, fish
- Peanuts
- Oats

Useful information

Because of their ability to maintain blood sugar levels, some doctors believe that BCAAs (with other nutrients) may be a more ideal source of energy than glucose in hospital patients who need intravenous feeding, especially as they decrease the rate of breakdown and utilization of other amino acids.

Valine supplements may help to reverse hepatic coma, in which patients with cirrhosis of the liver are suffering from increased amounts of ammonia and tryptophan or tyrosine in the brain. Valine helps to reduce brain levels of tryptophan and tyrosine by competing with them for entry into the brain. Because it can be converted to glucose, it also acts as a useful fuel for brain metabolism.

Chronic fatigue syndrome

Research suggests that some patients with chronic fatigue syndrome (also known as ME) may have excessive levels of tryptophan in their plasma. Free tryptophan in the brain is converted to serotonin, which promotes drowsiness and prepares the body for sleep. Persistently high levels of brain serotonin can lead to persistent fatigue.

In severe chronic fatigue syndrome, a small amount of activity leaves the patient feeling as if he/she has done much more. This disease is still very poorly understood, and this sensation may be because the metabolism behaves as if the body has over-exercised. (We know, for instance, that lactic acid levels are often high in chronic fatigue syndrome, whereas in normal individuals they would be high only after much exertion).

In normal individuals, exertion reduces levels of the branched-chain amino acids, which compete with tryptophan for entry into the brain. This allows larger than usual amounts of tryptophan to enter the brain, where they are converted to serotonin, and promote drowsiness and fatigue. Supplementation with branched-chain amino acids may therefore help to combat excessive tryptophan levels in chronic fatigue sufferers[1]. It is also important for them to avoid consuming high-carbohydrate meals, which encourage tryptophan uptake into the brain.

SUPPLEMENTS

How to use valine supplements

Valine supplements are usually available only in combined BCAA products.

BCAA supplements are indicated for any form of physical stress and for the healing of severe wounds and injuries. Suggested regimes are 2-4 grams per day of leucine and 1-2 grams each of isoleucine and valine, taken:

- During intensive athletic training
- In chronic fatigue syndrome
- For up to a week before and after participating in a major athletic event
- Plus 1 gram vitamin C and 20 mg zinc, taken as needed after a major injury or fever
- Plus 1 gram vitamin C and 20 mg zinc, taken for up to a week before and two weeks after surgery.

For non-vegetarian athletes, gelatine, which can be stirred into soups and made into jelly with fruit juice, is an ideal supplement as it is cheap and extremely rich in branched-chain amino acids but contains no tryptophan. Foods rich in BCAAs should also be consumed.

How safe are valine supplements?

BCAAs compete with each other and with tyrosine, phenylalanine, tryptophan and methionine for transport to the brain, so exceptionally high levels of BCAAs (as in intravenous feeding) could lead to a decrease in the brain of the important chemicals serotonin and dopamine, which are made from these amino acids.

Valine content of common foods in grams per 100 g

Gelatine, dry	2.08
Cheese, cheddar	1.66
Sunflower seeds, hulled	1.32
Tuna, skipjack, fresh, raw	1.13
Chicken meat, raw	1.06
Salmon, Atlantic, farmed, raw	1.03
Pork, composite of various cuts, trimmed, raw	1.02
Peanuts, dry roasted	0.99
Prawns, boiled	0.98
Oats	0.94
Herring, Atlantic, raw	0.93
Brazil nuts, raw	0.91
Beef, ground, extra-lean (approx. 21% fat)	0.86
Almonds, raw	0.80
Eggs, hard-boiled	0.77
Walnuts, raw	0.75
Buckwheat flour, whole groat	0.65
Wheat flour, whole-grain	0.62
Lentils, boiled	0.45
Yoghurt, plain, low-fat	0.43
Cornmeal, whole-grain, yellow	0.41
Tofu, raw, with calcium sulphate	0.41
Chick peas, boiled	0.37
Beans, baked	0.25
Rice, brown, long-grain, boiled	0.15
Broccoli, boiled, drained	0.14
Mushrooms, raw	0.13
Avocados, raw	0.10
Potatoes, peeled, boiled	0.10
Beetroot (beets) boiled, drained	0.06
Bananas, raw	0.05
Apricots, raw	0.05
Carrots, boiled, drained	0.05
Aubergine (eggplant) boiled, drained	0.04
Cabbage, boiled, drained	0.04
Oranges, raw	0.04
Peppers, sweet, green, raw	0.04
Onions, boiled, drained	0.03
Apples, raw with skin	0.01

Source: USDA National Nutrient Database for Standard Reference, Release 28

APPENDIX I

Amino Acids in

48 Common Foods

Grams per 100 g	Tryp to phan	Threo nine	Isoleu cine	Leu cine	Ly sine	Me thio nine	Cys tine	Phe nyla lanine	Tyro sine	Va line	Argi nine	Histi dine	Ala nine	Aspar tic acid	Gluta mic acid	Gly cine	Pro line	Se rine
Almonds, raw	0.19	0.68	0.69	1.47	0.60	0.19	0.28	1.15	0.53	0.80	2.47	0.59	1.00	2.73	5.17	1.47	0.97	1.01
Apples, raw with skin	0.00	0.01	0.01	0.01	0.01	0.00	0.00	0.01	0.00	0.01	0.01	0.00	0.01	0.03	0.02	0.01	0.01	0.01
Apricots, raw	0.02	0.05	0.04	0.08	0.10	0.01	0.00	0.05	0.03	0.05	0.05	0.03	0.07	0.31	0.16	0.04	0.10	0.08
Aubergine (eggplant) boiled, drained	0.01	0.03	0.04	0.05	0.04	0.01	0.00	0.04	0.02	0.04	0.05	0.02	0.04	0.13	0.15	0.03	0.03	0.03
Avocados, raw	0.02	0.07	0.07	0.12	0.09	0.04	0.02	0.07	0.05	0.10	0.06	0.03	0.12	0.28	0.21	0.08	0.08	0.08
Bananas, raw	0.01	0.03	0.03	0.07	0.05	0.01	0.02	0.04	0.02	0.05	0.05	0.08	0.04	0.11	0.11	0.04	0.04	0.05
Beans, baked	0.06	0.20	0.21	0.38	0.33	0.07	0.05	0.26	0.14	0.25	0.30	0.13	0.20	0.58	0.73	0.19	0.20	0.26
Beef, ground, extra lean (21% fat)	0.22	0.74	0.76	1.42	1.48	0.41	0.17	0.67	0.55	0.86	1.19	0.56	1.16	1.62	2.78	1.31	0.90	0.69
Beetroot (beets) boiled, drained	0.02	0.05	0.05	0.07	0.06	0.02	0.02	0.05	0.04	0.06	0.04	0.02	0.06	0.12	0.45	0.03	0.04	0.06
Brazil nuts, raw	0.26	0.46	0.60	1.19	0.54	1.01	0.35	0.75	0.46	0.91	2.39	0.40	0.57	1.36	3.15	0.66	0.76	0.75
Broccoli, boiled, drained	0.03	0.10	0.12	0.14	0.15	0.04	0.02	0.09	0.07	0.14	0.16	0.05	0.13	0.23	0.40	0.10	0.12	0.11
Buckwheat flour, whole groat	0.18	0.48	0.47	0.79	0.64	0.16	0.22	0.50	0.23	0.65	0.94	0.29	0.71	1.08	1.95	0.98	0.48	0.65
Butter beans (lima beans), boiled, drained	0.09	0.34	0.41	0.67	0.52	0.10	0.09	0.45	0.28	0.47	0.48	0.24	0.40	1.01	1.10	0.33	0.35	0.52
Cabbage, boiled, drained	0.01	0.04	0.05	0.05	0.05	0.01	0.01	0.03	0.02	0.04	0.06	0.02	0.04	0.10	0.22	0.02	0.20	0.06
Carrots, boiled, drained	0.01	0.04	0.04	0.05	0.04	0.01	0.01	0.03	0.02	0.05	0.05	0.02	0.06	0.14	0.21	0.03	0.03	0.04
Cheese, cheddar	0.32	0.89	1.55	2.39	2.07	0.65	0.13	1.31	1.20	1.66	0.94	0.87	0.70	1.60	6.09	0.43	2.81	1.46
Chick peas, boiled	0.09	0.33	0.38	0.63	0.59	0.12	0.12	0.48	0.22	0.37	0.84	0.24	0.38	1.04	1.55	0.37	0.37	0.45

Food																		
Chicken meat, raw	0.25	0.90	1.13	1.61	1.82	0.59	0.27	0.85	0.72	1.06	1.29	0.66	1.17	1.91	3.20	1.05	0.88	0.74
Cocoa powder, dry	0.29	0.78	0.76	1.19	0.98	0.20	0.24	0.94	0.74	1.18	1.11	0.34	0.90	1.95	2.95	0.88	0.84	0.85
Coconut meat, raw	0.04	0.12	0.13	0.25	0.15	0.06	0.07	0.17	0.10	0.20	0.55	0.08	0.17	0.33	0.76	0.16	0.14	0.17
Cornmeal, whole-grain, yellow	0.06	0.31	0.29	1.00	0.23	0.17	0.15	0.40	0.33	0.41	0.41	0.25	0.61	0.57	1.53	0.33	0.71	0.39
Dark chocolate	0.06	0.17	0.16	0.26	0.21	0.04	0.05	0.20	0.16	0.25	0.24	0.07	0.20	0.42	0.64	0.19	0.18	0.18
Eggs, hard-boiled	0.15	0.60	0.69	1.08	0.90	0.39	0.29	0.67	0.51	0.77	0.76	0.30	0.70	1.26	1.64	0.42	0.50	0.94
Gelatine, dry	0.00	1.48	1.16	2.45	3.46	0.61	0.00	1.74	0.30	2.08	6.62	0.66	8.01	5.27	8.75	19.05	12.30	2.61
Herring, Atlantic, raw	0.20	0.79	0.83	1.46	1.65	0.53	0.19	0.70	0.61	0.93	1.08	0.53	1.09	1.84	2.68	0.86	0.64	0.73
Lentils, boiled	0.08	0.32	0.39	0.65	0.63	0.08	0.12	0.45	0.24	0.45	0.70	0.25	0.38	1.00	1.40	0.37	0.38	0.42
Milk chocolate	0.08	0.30	0.37	0.65	0.41	0.15	0.04	0.38	0.32	0.45	0.20	0.11	0.24	0.58	1.45	0.17	0.58	0.32
Millet, boiled	0.04	0.11	0.15	0.45	0.07	0.07	0.07	0.19	0.11	0.18	0.12	0.08	0.31	0.23	0.76	0.09	0.28	0.21
Mung beans, boiled, drained	0.08	0.23	0.30	0.54	0.49	0.08	0.06	0.43	0.21	0.36	0.49	0.21	0.31	0.81	1.26	0.28	0.32	0.35
Mushrooms, raw	0.07	0.13	0.12	0.18	0.29	0.06	0.01	0.11	0.06	0.13	0.14	0.08	0.22	0.27	0.50	0.13	0.20	0.13
Oats	0.23	0.58	0.69	1.28	0.70	0.31	0.41	0.90	0.57	0.94	1.19	0.41	0.88	1.45	3.71	0.84	0.93	0.75
Onions, boiled, drained	0.02	0.03	0.05	0.05	0.07	0.01	0.02	0.04	0.03	0.03	0.18	0.02	0.04	0.07	0.22	0.06	0.04	0.04
Oranges, raw	0.01	0.02	0.03	0.02	0.05	0.02	0.01	0.03	0.02	0.04	0.07	0.02	0.05	0.11	0.09	0.09	0.05	0.03
Peanuts, dry roasted	0.23	0.81	0.83	1.54	0.85	0.29	0.30	1.23	0.96	0.99	2.83	0.60	0.94	2.89	4.95	1.43	1.05	1.17
Peas, green, boiled, drained	0.04	0.20	0.19	0.32	0.31	0.08	0.03	0.20	0.11	0.23	0.42	0.11	0.24	0.49	0.73	0.18	0.17	0.18
Peppers, sweet, green, raw	0.01	0.03	0.03	0.05	0.04	0.01	0.02	0.03	0.02	0.04	0.04	0.02	0.04	0.13	0.12	0.03	0.04	0.04
Pork, composite of cuts, trimmed, raw	0.23	0.86	0.87	1.51	1.70	0.49	0.24	0.75	0.65	1.02	1.20	0.74	1.11	1.74	2.92	0.98	0.81	0.78
Potatoes, peeled, boiled	0.03	0.06	0.07	0.10	0.10	0.03	0.02	0.08	0.06	0.10	0.08	0.04	0.05	0.42	0.29	0.05	0.06	0.08

Prawns, boiled	0.29	0.85	1.01	1.66	1.82	0.59	0.23	0.88	0.70	0.98	1.83	0.43	1.18	2.16	3.57	1.26	0.69	0.82
Pumpkin, boiled, drained	0.01	0.02	0.02	0.03	0.04	0.01	0.00	0.02	0.03	0.03	0.04	0.01	0.02	0.07	0.13	0.02	0.02	0.03
Rice, brown, long-grain, boiled	0.03	0.10	0.11	0.21	0.10	0.06	0.03	0.13	0.10	0.15	0.20	0.07	0.15	0.24	0.53	0.13	0.12	0.13
Salmon, Atlantic, farmed, raw	0.22	0.87	0.92	1.62	1.83	0.59	0.21	0.78	0.67	1.03	1.19	0.59	1.20	2.04	2.97	0.96	0.70	0.81
Sunflower seeds, hulled	0.35	0.93	1.14	1.66	0.94	0.49	0.45	1.17	0.67	1.32	2.40	0.63	1.12	2.45	5.58	1.46	1.18	1.08
Tofu, raw, with calcium sulphate	0.13	0.33	0.40	0.61	0.53	0.10	0.11	0.39	0.27	0.41	0.54	0.24	0.33	0.89	1.40	0.32	0.44	0.38
Tuna, skipjack, fresh, raw	0.25	0.96	1.01	1.79	2.02	0.65	0.24	0.86	0.74	1.13	1.32	0.65	1.33	2.25	3.28	1.06	0.78	0.90
Walnuts, raw	0.17	0.60	0.63	1.17	0.42	0.24	0.21	0.71	0.41	0.75	2.28	0.39	0.70	1.83	2.82	0.82	0.71	0.93
Wheat flour, whole-grain	0.21	0.40	0.51	0.93	0.38	0.21	0.32	0.65	0.40	0.62	0.64	0.32	0.49	0.70	4.33	0.55	1.42	0.65
Yoghurt, plain, low-fat	0.03	0.22	0.29	0.53	0.47	0.16	0.05	0.29	0.27	0.43	0.16	0.13	0.23	0.42	1.03	0.13	0.62	0.33

Data Source

USDA National Nutrient Database for Standard Reference, Release 28

REFERENCES

to sources of

scientific information

Alanine

1. Stumvoll, Michael, et al. Glutamine and Alanine Metabolism in Non-Insulin-Dependent Diabetes Mellitus. Diabetes, July, 1996;45:863-868. University of Rochester, New York, USA.

2. Hoffman J, Ratamess NA et al. Beta-alanine and the hormonal response to exercise. Int J Sports Med. 2008 Dec;29 (12):952-8.

3. Walter AA, Smith AE et al. Six weeks of high-intensity interval training with and without beta-alanine supplementation for improving cardiovascular fitness in women. J Strength Cond Res. 2010 May;24(5):1199-207.

4. Gross M, Boesch C et al. Effects of beta-alanine supplementation and interval training on physiological determinants of severe exercise performance. Eur J Appl Physiol. 2014 Feb;114(2):221-34.

5. Ducker KJ, Dawson B et al. Effect of beta-alanine supplementation on 800-m running performance. Int J Sport Nutr Exerc Metab. 2013 Dec;23(6):554-61.

6. Gross M, Bieri K et al. Beta-alanine supplementation improves jumping power and affects severe-intensity performance in professional alpine skiers. Int J Sport Nutr Exerc Metab. 2014 Dec;24(6):665-73.

7. McCormack WP, Stout JR et al. Oral nutritional supplement fortified with beta-alanine improves physical working capacity in older adults: a randomized, placebo-controlled study. Exp Gerontol. 2013 Sep;48(9):933-9.

8. Hoffman JR, Stout JR et al. β-Alanine supplementation and military performance. Amino Acids. 2015 Dec;47 (12):2463-74.

9. Trexler ET, Smith-Ryan AE et al. International society of sports nutrition position stand: Beta-Alanine. J Int Soc Sports Nutr. 2015 Jul 15;12:30.

Arginine

1. Siani A, Pagano E et al. Institute of Food Sciences and Technology, National Research Council, Avellino, Italy. Blood pressure and metabolic changes during dietary L-arginine supplementation in humans. American Journal of Hypertension 2000 May;13(5 Pt 1):547-51.

2. Chang CK, Chang Chien KM et al. Branched-chain amino acids and arginine improve performance in two consecutive days of simulated handball games in male and female athletes: a randomized trial. PLoS One. 2015 Mar 24;10(3).

3. Camic CL, Housh TJ et al. Effects of arginine-based supplements on the physical working capacity at the fatigue threshold. J Strength Cond Res. 2010 May;24(5):1306-12.

4. Bednarz B, Jaxa-Chamiec T et al. L-arginine supplementation prolongs exercise capacity in congestive heart failure. Kardiol Pol. 2004 Apr;60(4):348-53.

5. Bogdanski P, Suliburska J et al. Effect of 3-month L-arginine supplementation on insulin resistance and tumor necrosis factor activity in patients with visceral obesity. Eur Rev Med Pharmacol Sci. 2012 Jun;16(6):816-23.

6. Suliburska J, Bogdanski P et al. Changes in mineral status are associated with improvements in insulin sensitivity in obese patients following L-arginine supplementation. Eur J Nutr. 2014;53(2):387-93.

7. Dashtabi A, Mazloom Z et al. Oral L-Arginine Administration Improves Anthropometric and Biochemical Indices

Associated With Cardiovascular Diseases in Obese Patients: A Randomized, Single Blind Placebo Controlled Clinical Trial. Research in Cardiovascular Medicine. 2016;5(1).
8. Fayh AP, Krause M et al. Effects of L-arginine supplementation on blood flow, oxidative stress status and exercise responses in young adults with uncomplicated type I diabetes. Eur J Nutr. 2013 Apr;52(3):975-83.
9. Cherla G1, Jaimes EA. Role of L-arginine in the pathogenesis and treatment of renal disease. J Nutr. 2004 Oct;134(10 Suppl):2801S-2806S; discussion 2818S-2819S.
10. Wu G, Meininger CJ . Arginine Nutrition and Cardiovascular Function. J Nutr, 2000;130:2626-2629. Dept Animal Sci and Faculty of Nutr, Texas A&M Univ, USA.
11. Chuman H, Chuman T, Nao-i N, Sawada A. Department of Ophthalmology, Miyazaki Medical College, Miyazaki, Japan. The effect of L-arginine on intraocular pressure in the human eye. Current Eye Research 2000 Jun;20 (6):511-6.
12. Reyes AA, Karl IE, Klahr S. Role of arginine in health and in renal disease. Am J Physiol 1994 Sep;267(3 Pt 2):F331-46.
13. Yatzidis H. Oral supplement of six selective amino acids arrest progression renal failure in uremic patients. Int Urol Nephrol. 2004;36(4):591-8.
14. Ohtsuka Y, Nakaya J. Effect of oral administration of L-arginine on senile dementia. American Journal of Medicine 2000;108:439.
15. Loukides, S, et al. Effect of Arginine on Mucociliary Function in Primary Ciliary Dyskinesia. Lancet, August 1, 1998;352:371-372. Department of Thoracic Medicine, Im-

perial College School of Medicine at the National Heart and Lung Institute, London, United Kingdom.

16. Chigo E, Ceda GP, Valcavi R, et al. Low doses of either intravenously or orally administered arginine are able to enhance growth hormone response to growth hormone releasing hormone in elderly subjects. J Endocrinol Invest 1994; 17:113-117.

17. Elam RP. Morphological changes in adult males from resistance exercise and amino acid supplementation. Journal of Sports Medicine and Physical Fitness 1998;28:35-9.

18. Tan B, Li X et al. Regulatory roles for L-arginine in reducing white adipose tissue. Front Biosci (Landmark Ed). 2012 Jun 1;17:2237-46.

19. Hristina K, Langerholc T et al. Novel metabolic roles of L-arginine in body energy metabolism and possible clinical applications. J Nutr Health Aging. 2014;18(2):213-8.

20. Monti LD, Setola E et al. Effect of a long-term oral l-arginine supplementation on glucose metabolism: a randomized, double-blind, placebo-controlled trial. Diabetes Obes Metab. 2012 Oct;14(10):893-900.

21. Appleton J. Arginine: Clinical potential of a semi-essential amino acid. Altern Med Rev. 2002 Dec;7(6):512-22.

22. Zhu Q, Yue X et al. Effect of L-arginine supplementation on blood pressure in pregnant women: a meta-analysis of placebo-controlled trials. Hypertens Pregnancy. 2013;32 (1):32-41.

23. Kang K, Shu XL et al. Effect of L-arginine on immune function: a meta-analysis. Asia Pac J Clin Nutr. 2014;23 (3):351-9.

24. Grimble GK. Adverse gastrointestinal effects of argin-

ine and related amino acids. J Nutr. 2007 Jun;137(6 Suppl 2):1693S-1701S.
25. Park KG1, Heys SD et al. Stimulation of human breast cancers by dietary L-arginine. Clin Sci (Lond). 1992 Apr;82(4):413-7.
26. Brittenden J1, Park KG et al. L-arginine stimulates host defenses in patients with breast cancer. Surgery. 1994 Feb;115(2):205-12.

Aspartate

1. Trudeau F. Aspartate as an ergogenic supplement. Sports Med. 2008;38(1):9-16.

Carnitine

1. Jacob C, Belleville F. Laboratoire de Biochimie B-CHRU Nancy, France. L-carnitine: metabolism, functions and value in pathology. [Article in French] Pathol Biol (Paris) 1992 Nov;40(9):910-9.
2. Krahenbuhl S. L-carnitine and vegetarianism. Annals of Nutrition and Metabolism 2000;44:81-81.
3. Plioplys AV, Plioplys S. Chronic Fatigue Syndrome Center, Department of Research, Mercy Hospital Chicago, Ill 60616, USA. Amantadine and L-carnitine treatment of Chronic Fatigue Syndrome. Neuropsychobiology 1997;35 (1):16-23.
4. Davini P, Bigalli A, Lamanna F, Boem A. Controlled study on L-carnitine therapeutic efficacy in post-infarction. *Drugs Exp Clin Res.* 1992;18(8):355-65.
5. Bartels GL, Remme WJ et al. Sticares Cardiovascular Research Foundation, Zuiderziekenhuis, Rotterdam, The Netherlands. Effects of L-propionylcarnitine on ischemia-

induced myocardial dysfunction in men with angina pectoris. Am J Cardiol 1994 Jul 15;74(2):125-30.

6. 11. Hiatt WR, Regensteiner JG, Creager MA, et al. Propionyl-L-Carnitine Improves Exercise Performance and Functional Status in Patients With Claudication. Am J Med, June 1, 2001;110:616-622. University of Colorado Health Sciences Center, Denver, Colorado USA.

7. Colonna P, Iliceto S. Institute of Cardiology, University of Cagliari, Italy. Myocardial infarction and left ventricular remodeling: results of the CEDIM trial. Carnitine Ecocardiografia Digitalizzata Infarto Miocardico. Am Heart J 2000 Feb;139(2 Pt 3):S124-30.

8. Anand I, Chandrashekhan Y et al. VA Medical Center, Minneapolis, Minnesota, USA. Acute and chronic effects of propionyl-L-carnitine on the hemodynamics, exercise capacity, and hormones in patients with congestive heart failure. Cardiovasc Drugs Ther 1998 Jul;12(3):291-9.

9. Pettegrew JW, Levine J, McClure RJ. Department of Psychiatry, School of Medicine, University of Pittsburgh, USA. Acetyl-L-carnitine physical-chemical, metabolic, and therapeutic properties: relevance for its mode of action in Alzheimer's disease and geriatric depression. Mol Psychiatry 2000 Nov;5(6):616-32.

10. Carta A, Calvani M. Acetyl-L-Carnitine: A Drug Able to Slow the Progress of Alzheimer's Disease?'. Ann NY Acad Sci, 1991;640:228-232.

11. Salvioli G, Neri M. L-acetylcarnitine treatment of mental decline in the elderly. *Drugs Exp Clin Res.* 1994;20 (4):169-76.

12. Schaffhauser AO, Gaynor PT. L-Carnitine Supplementation-A Natural Approach for Weight Management. Ann

Nutr Metab, 2000;44:94-95.

13. Wutzke KD, Lorenz H. The effect of l-carnitine on fat oxidation, protein turnover, and body composition in slightly overweight subjects. *Metabolism.* 2004 Aug;53 (8):1002-6.

14. Huang A, Owen K Role of supplementary L-carnitine in exercise and exercise recovery. Med Sport Sci. 2012;59:135-42.

15. Kraemer WJ, Volek JS et al. L-carnitine supplementation: influence upon physiological function. Curr Sports Med Rep. 2008 Jul-Aug;7(4):218-23.

16. Cavallini G, Ferraretti AP et al. Cinnoxicam and L-carnitine/acetyl-L-carnitine treatment for idiopathic and varicocele-associated oligoasthenospermia. *J Androl.* 2004 Sep-Oct;25(5):761-70; discussion 71-2.

17. Benvenga S, Amato A et al. Effects of carnitine on thyroid hormone action. Ann NY Acad Sci. 2004 Nov;1033:158-67.

18. Seidman MD, Khan MJ, et al. Biologic Acitivity of Mitochondrial Metabolites on Aging and Age-Related Hearing Loss. The American Journal of Otology, 2000; 21: 161-167.

19. Coleman JKM, Kopke RD, et al. Pharmacological Rescue of Noise Induced Hearing Loss Using N-Acetylcysteine and Acetyl-L-Carnitine. Hearing Research, 2007; 226: 104-113.

20. Dodson WL, Sachan DS. Department of Nutrition, University of Tennessee, Knoxville 37996-1900, USA. Choline supplementation reduces urinary carnitine excretion in humans. Am J Clin Nutr 1996 Jun;63(6):904-10 Comment in: Am J Clin Nutr. 1997 Feb;65(2):574-9.

Cysteine

1. Breitkreutz R, Pittack N et al. Deutsches Krebsforschungszentrum, Division of Immunochemistry, Heidelberg, Germany. Improvement of immune functions in HIV infection by sulfur supplementation: two randomized trials. J Mol Med 2000;78(1):55-62. Comment in: J Mol Med. 2000 ;78(1):1-2.
2. Unoki H, Bujo H et al. Advanced glycation end products attenuate cellular insulin sensitivity by increasing the generation of intracellular reactive oxygen species in adipocytes. Diabetes Res Clin Pract. 2007 May;76(2):236-44.
3. Stey C, Steurer J et al. Dept of Internal Medicine, Medical Polyclinic, University Hospital Zurich, Switzerland. The effect of oral n-acetyl cysteine in chronic bronchitis: a quantitative systematic review. Eur Respir J 2000 Aug;16 (2):253-62.
4. De Benedetto F, Aceto A et al. Long-term oral n-acetyl cysteine reduces exhaled hydrogen peroxide in stable COPD. Pulm Pharmacol Ther. 2005;18(1):41-7.
5. Stav D, Raz M. Effect of n-acetyl cysteine on air trapping in COPD: a randomized placebo-controlled study. Chest. 2009 Aug;136(2):381-6.
6. Geiler J, Michaelis M et al. N-acetyl-L-cysteine (NAC) inhibits virus replication and expression of pro-inflammatory molecules in A549 cells infected with highly pathogenic H5N1 influenza A virus. Biochem Pharmacol. 2010 Feb 1;79(3):413-20.
7. Albini A, D'Agostini F et al. Istituto Nazionale per la Ricerca sul Cancro, Genoa, Italy. Inhibition of invasion, gelatinase activity, tumor take and metastasis of malignant cells by n-acetyl cysteine. Int J Cancer 1995 Mar 29;61

(1):121-9.

8. Conklin KA. Dietary Antioxidants During Cancer Chemotherapy: Impact on Chemotherapeutic Effectiveness and Development of Side Effects. Nutrition and Cancer, 2000;37(1):1-18. Los Angeles School of Medicine, University of California, USA.

9. Ovesen T, Felding JU et al. ENT Department, Aarhus University Hospital, Denmark. Effect of n-acetyl cysteine on the incidence of recurrence of otitis media with effusion and re-insertion of ventilation tubes. Acta Otolaryngol Suppl 2000;543:79-81.

10. Lindblad AC, Rosenhall U et al. The efficacy of n-acetyl cysteine to protect the human cochlea from subclinical hearing loss caused by impulse noise: A controlled trial. Noise Health. 2011 Nov-Dec;13(55):392-401.

11. Lin CY, Wu JL et al. N-Acetyl-cysteine against noise-induced temporary threshold shift in male workers. Hear Res. 2010 Oct 1;269(1-2):42-7.

12. Salim AS. University Department of Surgery, Medical City, Baghdad, Iraq. Sulphydryl-containing agents and the prevention of duodenal ulcer relapse. Pharmacology 1993 May;46(5):281-8.

13. Fulghesu AM, Ciampelli M et al. N-acetyl-cysteine treatment improves insulin sensitivity in women with polycystic ovary syndrome. Fertil Steril. 2002 Jun;77(6):1128-35.

14. Masha A, Manieri C et al. Prolonged treatment with n-acetyl cysteine and L-arginine restores gonadal function in patients with PCO syndrome. J Endocrinol Invest. 2009 Apr 15.

15. Oner G, Muderris II. Clinical, endocrine and metabolic

effects of metformin vs. N-acetyl-cysteine in women with polycystic ovary syndrome. Euro 1 Obstet Gynecol Reprod Biol. 2011;159(1):127-131.

16. Berk M, et al. n-acetyl cysteine for depressive symptoms in bipolar disorder-a double-blind randomized placebo-controlled trial. Biol Psychiatry. 2008;64:468-475.

17. Bounous G. Cancer and whey protein. Clinical Pearls News 2001 Oct;ll(10):161.

18. Lands LC, Grey VL, Smountas AA. Division of Respiratory Medicine, McGill University Health Centre-Montreal Children's Hospital, Montreal, Quebec, Canada H3H 1P3. Effect of supplementation with a cysteine donor on muscular performance. J Appl Physiol 1999 Oct;87 (4):1381-5 Erratum in: J Appl Physiol 2000 Jan;88(1).

19. Bounous G. Whey protein concentrate (WPC) and glutathione modulation in cancer treatment. Anticancer Research 2000;20:4785-92.

GABA

1. Kakuda T. Neuroprotective effects of theanine and its preventive effects on cognitive dysfunction. Pharmacol Res. 2011 Aug;64(2):162-8.

2. Cases J et al. Pilot trial of Melissa officinalis L. leaf extract in the treatment of volunteers suffering from mild-tomoderate anxiety disorders and sleep disturbances. Med I Nutrition Metab. 2011 Dec;4(3):211-218.

3. Franco L et al. The sedative effects of hops (Humulus lupulus), a component of beer, on the activity/rest rhythm. Acta Phys Hung. 2012 Jun;99(2):133-139.

4. Braverman ER. The Healing Nutrients Within. Keats Publishing Inc., New Canaan, USA, 1997.

Glutamine

1. Zuhl M, Dokladny K et al. The effects of acute oral glutamine supplementation on exercise-induced gastrointestinal permeability and heat shock protein expression in peripheral blood mononuclear cells. Cell Stress Chaperones. 2015 Jan;20(1):85-93.

2. Munro HN, Crim MC: The proteins and amino acids. In Eds Shils ME and Young VR: Modern Nutrition in Health and Diseases. Lea & Febiger, Philadelphia, 1988, pp 1-37.

3. Rogers LL, Pelton RB. Glutamine in the treatment of alcoholism. Q J Stud Alcohol 18(4):581-7, 1957.

4. Jukić T, Rojc B et al. The use of a food supplementation with D-phenylalanine, L-glutamine and L-5-hydroxytriptophan in the alleviation of alcohol withdrawal symptoms. Coll Antropol. 2011 Dec;35(4):1225-30.

5. Van Acker BA, von Meyenfeldt MF, Soeters PB. Academisch Ziekenhuis, afd. Algemene Chirurgie, Maastricht. Glutamine as a key ingredient in protein metabolism. [Article in Dutch] Ned Tijdschr Geneeskd 1999 Sep 18;143 (38):1904-8.

6. Miller AL. Therapeutic considerations of L-glutamine: a review of the literature. Altern Med Rev 1999 Aug;4 (4):239-48.

7. Hammarqvist F, Wernerman J et al. Addition of glutamine to total parenteral nutrition after elective abdominal surgery spares free glutamine in muscle, counteracts the fall in muscle protein synthesis, and improves nitrogen balance. Ann Surg. 1989 Apr;209(4):455-61.

8. Rubio IT, Cao Y et al. Department of Surgery, University of Arkansas for Medical Sciences, Little Rock 72205, USA. Effect of glutamine on methotrexate efficacy and

toxicity. Annals of Surgery 1998 May;227(5):772-8; discussion 778-80.

9. Kuhn KS, Muscaritoli M et al. Glutamine as indispensable nutrient in oncology: experimental and clinical evidence. Eur J Nutr. 2010;49:197-210.

10. Furukawa S et al. Glutamine-Enhanced Bacterial Killing by Neutrophils From Postoperative Patients. Nutrition, 1997;13(10):863-869.

11. Castell LM, Newsholme EA. University Department of Biochemistry, Oxford, United Kingdom. The relation between glutamine and the immunodepression observed in exercise. Amino Acids 2001;20(1):49-61.

12. Miller AL. Therapeutic considerations of L-glutamine: a review of the literature. Altern Med Rev. 1999 Aug;4 (4):239-48.

13. Welbourne TC. Increased plasma bicarbonate and growth hormone after an oral glutamine load. Am J Clin Nutr. 1995 May;61(5):1058-61.

14. Shao A, Hathcock JN. Risk assessment for the amino acids taurine, L-glutamine and L-arginine. Regul Toxicol Pharmacol. 2008 Apr;50(3):376-99.

Glutathione

1. Miller GW, Kirby ML et al. Heptachlor alters expression and function of dopamine transporters. Neurotoxicology 1999;20(4):631-7.

2. Sechi G, Deledda MG, Bua G, et al. Reduced Intravenous Glutathione in the Treatment of Early Parkinson's Disease. Prog Neuro-Psychopharmacol & Biol Psychiat, 1996;20:1159-1170.

3. Cheney, P. Clinical management of chronic fatigue syn-

drome. Transcription on internet website of lecture dated 5-7 February 1999. www.nutritionadvisor.com/cheneymd.html.

4. Nathan N, Van Konynenburg RA. Treatment study of patients with chronic fatigue syndrome and fibromyalgia, based on the glutathione depletion--methylation cycle block hypothesis. Townsend Lett. Dec 2011:53-59.

5. Packer L. The Antioxidant Miracle. John Wiley & Sons Inc., Chichester, 1999.

6. Passwater RA. Antioxidant Cocktail Update: Part 2 Lesser known antioxidant are very important. An Interview with Dr. Lester Packer. Whole Foods magazine, November 1999.

7. Vendemiale G, Altomare E et al. Effects of oral S-adenosyl-L-methionine on hepatic glutathione in patients with liver disease. Scand J Gastroenterol. 1989 May;24 (4):407-15.

8. Basu A, Betts NM et al. Green tea supplementation increases glutathione and plasma antioxidant capacity in adults with the metabolic syndrome. Nutr Res. 2013 Mar;33(3):180-7.

9. Jain A, Buist NR et al. Effect of ascorbate or n-acetyl cysteine treatment in a patient with hereditary glutathione synthetase deficiency. J Pediatr. 1994 Feb;124(2):229-33.

10. Durgaprasad S, Pai CG et al. A pilot study of the anti-oxidant effect of curcumin in tropical pancreatitis. Indian J Med Res. 2005 Oct;122(4):315-8.

Glycine Reference

1. Braverman ER. The Healing Nutrients Within. Keats Publishing Inc., New Canaan, USA, 1997.

2. Aito K, Iwatsubo E. [The conservative treatment of prostatic hypertrophy with Paraprost.] [in Japanese] Hinyokika Kiyo 18(1):41-4, 1972.

3. Heresco-Levy U, et al. Efficacy of High-Dose Glycine in the Treatment of Enduring Negative Symptoms of Schizophrenia. Arch Gen Psychiatry, January, 1999;56:29-36. Ezrath Nashim-Herzog Memorial Hospital, Jerusalem, Israel.

4. Ishimaru MJ, Toru, M. The Glutamate Hypothesis of Schizophrenia: Therapeutic Implications. CNS Drugs, January, 1997;7(1):47-67. Department of Psychiatry, Washington University School of Medicine, St. Louis, USA.

5. Brunk D. Gelatin Supplement May Help Arthritic Knees. Family Practice News, December 1, 2000:12.

6. Yamadera W, Inagawa K et al. Glycine ingestion improves subjective sleep quality in human volunteers, correlating with polysomnographic changes. Sleep and Biological Rhythms. 2007;5(2):126-31.

7. Bolman WM, Richmond JA. A double-blind,placebo-controlled, crossover pilot trial of low dose dimethylglycine in patients with autistic disorder. J Autism Dev Disord 1999;29:191-194.

Histidine

1. Pinals RS et al. Treatment of rheumatoid arthritis with L-histidine: A randomized, placebo controlled, double-blind trial. Journal of Rheumatology 4(4):414-9, 1977.

2. Sadowska-Krowicka H et al. Reduction in Non-Steroidal

Anti- Inflammatory Drug-Induced Gastritis by Histidine. JANA, Winter, 1999;2(1):19-24. Dept. of Pediatrics, Albany Medical College, New York USA.

3. Yatzidis H. Oral supplement of six selective amino acids arrest progression renal failure in uremic patients. Int Urol Nephrol. 2004;36(4):591-8.

4. Feng RN1, Niu YC et al. Histidine supplementation improves insulin resistance through suppressed inflammation in obese women with the metabolic syndrome: a randomized controlled trial. Diabetologia. 2013 May;56(5):985-94.

5. Hipkiss AR. Carnosine and its possible roles in nutrition and health. Adv Food Nutr Res. 2009;57:87-154.

Isoleucine

1. Braverman ER. The Healing Nutrients Within. Keats Publishing Inc., New Canaan, USA, 1997.

2. Castell LM, Yamamoto T, Phoenix J, Newsholme EA. University Department of Biochemistry, Oxford, UK. The role of tryptophan in fatigue in different conditions of stress. Adv Exp Med Biol 1999;467:697-704.

Leucine

1. De Bandt JP1, Cynober L. Therapeutic use of branched-chain amino acids in burn, trauma, and sepsis. J Nutr. 2006 Jan;136(1 Suppl):308S-13S.

2. Verreijen AM1, Verlaan S1 et al. A high whey protein-, leucine-, and vitamin D-enriched supplement preserves muscle mass during intentional weight loss in obese older adults: a double-blind randomized controlled trial. Am J Clin Nutr. 2015 Feb;101(2):279-86.

3. Jitomir J1, Willoughby DS. Leucine for retention of lean

mass on a hypocaloric diet. J Med Food. 2008 Dec;11 (4):606-9.

4. Fujita S, Dreyer HC et al. Nutrient signalling in the regulation of human muscle protein synthesis. J Physiol. 2007 Jul 15;582(Pt 2):813-23.

5. Dreyer HC, Drummond MJ et al. Leucine-enriched essential amino acid and carbohydrate ingestion following resistance exercise enhances mTOR signaling and protein synthesis in human muscle. Am J Physiol Endocrinol Metab. 2008 Feb;294(2):E392–400.

6. Katsanos CS, Kobayashi H et al. A high proportion of leucine is required for optimal stimulation of the rate of muscle protein synthesis by essential amino acids in the elderly. Am J Physiol Endocrinol Metab. 2006 Aug;291 (2):E381–7.

7. Walker TB1, Smith J et al. The influence of 8 weeks of whey-protein and leucine supplementation on physical and cognitive performance. Int J Sport Nutr Exerc Metab. 2010 Oct;20(5):409-17.

8. Castell LM, Yamamoto T et al. University Department of Biochemistry, Oxford, UK. The role of tryptophan in fatigue in different conditions of stress. Adv Exp Med Biol 1999;467:697-704.

9. Mero A. Leucine Supplementation and Intensive Training. Sports Med, June, 1999;27(6):347-358.

10. Yang Y1, Wu Z et al. L-Leucine and NO-mediated cardiovascular function. Amino Acids. 2015 Mar;47(3):435-47.

11. Cynober L1, Bier DM et al. A proposal for an upper limit of leucine safe intake in healthy adults. J Nutr. 2012 Dec;142(12):2249S-2250S.

Lysine

1. Atanassova SS. Influence of the lysine on the calcium oxalate renal calculi. Int Urol Nephrol. 2014 Mar;46 (3):593-7.
2. Civitelli R, Villareal DT et al. Institute of Medical Pathology, University of Siena, Italy. Dietary L-lysine and calcium metabolism in humans. Nutrition 1992 Nov-Dec;8 (6):400-5.
3. Walsh DE et al: Subjective response to lysine in the therapy of herpes simplex. Journal of Antimicrobial Chemotherapy 12(5):489-96, 1983.
4. Griffith RS, Walsh DE, Myrmel KH, et al. Success of L-lysine Therapy in Frequently Recurrent Herpes Simplex Infection. Treatment and Prophylaxis. Dermatologica, 1987;175(4):183-190.
5. Smriga M1, Ando T et al. Oral treatment with L-lysine and L-arginine reduces anxiety and basal cortisol levels in healthy humans. Biomed Res. 2007 Apr;28(2):85-90.
6. Lakhan SE1, Vieira KF. Nutritional and herbal supplements for anxiety and anxiety-related disorders: systematic review. Nutr J. 2010 Oct 7;9:42.
7. Rath, M. The Process of Eradicating Heart Disease Has Become Irreversible. Journal of Applied Nutrition, 1996;48 (1 & 2):22-33.

Methionine

1. Rea W. Chemical Sensitivity Volume I. Lewis Publishers, Boca Raton, USA, 1992.
2. Braverman ER. The Healing Nutrients Within. Keats Publishing Inc., New Canaan, USA, 1997.
3. Meininger V, Flamier A et al. [L-Methionine treatment

of Parkinson's disease: preliminary results]. [Article in French] Rev Neurol (Paris) 1982;138(4):297-303.

4. Papakostas GI, Cassiello CF et al. Folates and S-adenosylmethionine for major depressive disorder. Can J Psychiatry. 2012 Jul;57(7):406-13.

5. De Vanna M, Rigamonti R. Oral S-Adenosyl-L-Methionine in Depression. Curr Ther Res, September 1992;52(3):478-485.

6. Bressa GM. S-Adenosyl-l-Methionine (SAMe) as Anti-depressant: Meta-Analysis of Clinical Studies. Acta Neurol Scand, 1994;154(Suppl.):7-14.

7. Bertolo RF, McBreairty LE. The nutritional burden of methylation reactions. Curr Opin Clin Nutr Metab Care. 2013 Jan;16:102-8.

8. Chan A, Tchantchou F et al. Dietary and genetic compromise in folate availability reduces acetylcholine, cognitive performance and increases aggression: critical role of S-adenosylmethionine. J Nutr Health Aging. 2008 Apr;12 (4):252-61.

9. Reynolds EH, Godfrey P et al. S-adenosylmethionine and Alzheimer's disease. Neurology 1989;39(Suppl 1):397/ Abstract 10.

10. Panza F, Frisardi V et al. Polyunsaturated fatty acid and S-adenosyl-methionine supplementation in predementia syndromes and Alzheimer's disease: a review. Scientific-WorldJournal. 2009 May 22;9:373-89.

11. Tchantchou F, Graves M et al. S-adenosylmethionine mediates glutathione efficacy by increasing glutathione S-transferase activity: implications for S-adenosyl methionine as a neuroprotective dietary supplement. J Alzheimers Dis. 2008 Jul;14(3):323-8.

12. Shea TB, Chan A. S-adenosyl methionine: a natural therapeutic agent effective against multiple hallmarks and risk factors associated with Alzheimer's disease. J Alzheimers Dis. 2008 Feb;13:67-70.13.

13. Suchy J, Lee S et al. Dietary supplementation with S-adenosyl methionine delays the onset of motor neuron pathology in a murine model of amyotrophic lateral sclerosis. Neuromolecular Med. 2010 Mar;12:86-97.

14. Wang YC, Chiang EP. Low-dose methotrexate inhibits methionine S-adenosyltransferase in vitro and in vivo. Mol Med. 2012 May 9;18:423-32.

15. Santini D, Vincenzi B et al. S-adenosylmethionine (SAM) supplementation for treatment of chemotherapy-induced liver injury. Anticancer Res. 2003 Nov-Dec;23 (6D):5173-9.

16. Gatto G, Caleri D, Michelacci S, Sicuteri F. Analgesizing effect of a methyl donor (S-adenosylmethionine) in migraine: an open clinical trial. Int I Clin Pharmacol Res. 1986;6:15-17.

17. Chavez M. SAMe:S-adenosylmethionine. Am J Health-Syst Pharm 2000;57:119-123.

18. Guo T, Chang L et al. S-adenosyl-L-methionine for the treatment of chronic liver disease: a systematic review and meta-analysis. PLoS One. 2015 Mar 16;10(3):e0122124.

19. Shoob HD, Sargent RG et al. Dietary methionine is involved in the etiology of neural tube defect-affected pregnancies in humans. J Nutr. 2001 Oct;131(10):2653-8.

20. Di Rocco A, Rogers JD et al. Department of Neurology, Beth Israel Medical Center-Albert Einstein College of Medicine, New York, NY 10003, USA. S-Adenosyl-Methionine improves depression in patients with Parkin-

son's disease in an open-label clinical trial. Movement Disorders 2000 Nov;15(6):1225-9.

21. Smythies JR, Halsey JH. Treatment of Parkinson's disease with L-methionine. Southern Medical Journal 1984;77:1577.

Ornithine

1. Kokubo T, Ikeshima E et al. A randomized, double-masked, placebo-controlled crossover trial on the effects of L-ornithine on salivary cortisol and feelings of fatigue of flushers the morning after alcohol consumption. Biopsychosocial Medicine. 2013;7:6.

2. Ornithine alpha-ketoglutarate improves wound healing in severe burn patients: a prospective randomized double-blind trial versus isonitrogenous controls. Crit Care Med 2000 Jun;28(6):1772-6.

3. Zajac A, Poprzecki S et al. Arginine and ornithine supplementation increases growth hormone and insulin-like growth factor-1 serum levels after heavy-resistance exercise in strength-trained thletes. J Strength Cond Res. 2010 Apr;24(4):1082-90.

4. Miyake M, Kirisako T et al. Randomized controlled trial of the effects of L-ornithine on stress markers and sleep quality in healthy workers. Nutr J. 2014 Jun 3;13:53.

5. Elam RP. Morphological changes in adult males from resistance exercise and amino acid supplementation. Journal of Sports Medicine and Physical Fitness 1998;28:35-9.

6. Braverman ER. The Healing Nutrients Within. Keats Publishing Inc, New Canaan, USA, 1997.

Phenylalanine

1. Kitahara M. A precursor study of the indoleamine and catecholamine hypotheses of depression using the dietary tryptophan and tyrosine ratios. Journal of Orthomolecular Medicine 5(4):210-14, 1990).

2. Donzelle G, Bernard L et al. [Curing trial of complicated oncologic pain by D-phenylalanine (author's transl)]. Anesth Analg (Paris). 1981;38(11-12):655-8.

3. Kitade T, Odahara Y et al. Studies on the enhanced effect of acupuncture analgesia and acupuncture anesthesia by D-phenylalanine (2nd report)--schedule of administration and clinical effects in low back pain and tooth extraction. Acupunct Electrother Res. 1990;15(2):121-35.

4. Ehrenpreis S, Balagot RC, Myles S, et al. Further studies on the analgesic activity of D-phenylalanine in mice and humans. EL Way, Ed. Proceedings of the International Narcotic Research Club Convention, 1979:379-82.

5. Russell AL, McCarty MF. DL-phenylalanine markedly potentiates opiate analgesia—an example of nutrient/ pharmaceutical up-regulation of the endogenous analgesia system. Med Hypotheses. 2000 Oct;55(4):283-8.

6. Ballinger AB, Clark ML L-phenylalanine releases cholecystokinin (CCK) and is associated with reduced food intake in humans: evidence for a physiological role of CCK in control of eating. Metabolism 1994 Jun;43(6):735-8. Department of Gastroenterology, St Bartholomew's Hospital, West Smithfield, London, UK.

7. Blum K, Briggs AH et al. Enkephalinase inhibition: regulation of ethanol intake in genetically predisposed mice. Alcohol. 1987 Nov-Dec;4(6):449-56.

8. Downs B, Oscar-Berman M, Waite R, et al. Have We

Hatched the Addiction Egg: Reward Deficiency Syndrome Solution System™. Journal of genetic syndrome & gene therapy 2013;4(136):14318.

9. Beckmann H, Athen D, Olteanu M, Zimmer R. DL-phenylalanine versus imipramine: a double-blind controlled study. Arch Psychiatr Nervenkr 1979 Jul 4;227(1):49-58.

10. Cormane RH, Siddiqui AH et al. Phenylalanine and UVA light for the treatment of vitiligo. Arch Dermatol Res 1985;277(2):126-30.

Proline

1. Janusz M, Zabłocka A. Colostral proline-rich polypeptides--immunoregulatory properties and prospects of therapeutic use in Alzheimer's disease. Curr Alzheimer Res. 2010 Jun;7(4):323-33.

2. Boldogh I, Aguilera-Aguirre L et al. Colostrinin decreases hypersensitivity and allergic responses to common allergens. Int Arch Allergy Immunol. 2008;146(4):298-306.

3. Hayasaka S, Saito T et al. Clinical trials of vitamin B6 and proline supplementation for gyrate atrophy of the choroid and retina. British Journal of Ophthalmology 1985 Apr;69(4):283-90.

Serine

1. Perlmutter D. Functional Therapeutics in Neurodegenerative Disease. J Applied Nutr, 1999;51(1):3-15. www.BrainRecovery.com.

2. Kidd PM. A review of nutrients and botanicals in the integrative management of cognitive dysfunction. Altern Med Rev 1999 Jun;4(3):144-61.

3. Palmieri, G., et al., Double-blind controlled trial of phos-

phatidylserine in patients with senile mental deterioration. Clin. Trials J. 1987;24:73-83.

4. Delwaide PJ, et al. Double-blind randomized controlled study of phosphatidylserine in senile demented patients. Acta Neurol Scand 1986 Feb;73(2):136-40.

5. Cenacchi T, et al. Cognitive decline in the elderly: a double-blind, placebo-controlled multicenter study on efficacy of phosphatidylserine administration. Aging (Milano) 1993 Apr;5(2):123-33.

6. Crook TH et al, Memory Assessment Clinics, Bethesda, Maryland, USA. With the Venderbilt University School of Medicine, Nashville, Tennessee, Stanford University School of Medicine, Palo Alto, California, and Fidia Pharmaceutical Corporation of Italy. Effects of phosphatidylserine in age-associated memory impairment. Neurology 41:644-649, 1991.

7. Rosadini G et al. Phosphatidylserine: quantitative EEG effects in healthy volunteers. Neuropsychobiology 24:42-48, 1991.

8. Funfgeld EW, et al. Double-blind study with phosphatidylserine (PS) in parkinsonian patients with senile dementia of Alzheimer's type (SDAT). Prog Clin Biol Res 1989;317:1235-46.

9. The SMID Group. Phosphatidylserine in the treatment of clinically diagnosed Alzheimer's disease. J Neural Transm Suppl 1987;24:287-92.

10. Amenta F, et al. Treatment of cognitive dysfunction associated with Alzheimer's disease with cholinergic precursors. Ineffective treatments or inappropriate approaches? Mech Ageing Dev 2001 Nov;122(16):2025-40.

11. Heiss WD, et al. Activation PET as an instrument to

determine therapeutic efficacy in Alzheimer's disease. Ann N Y Acad Sci 1993 Sep 24;695:327-31.

12. Engel RR, Double-blind cross-over study of phosphatidylserine vs. placebo in patients with early dementia of the Alzheimer type. Eur Neuropsychopharmacol 1992 Jun;2 (2):149-55.

13. Crook T, et al. Effects of Phosphatidylserine in Alzheimer's Disease. Psychopharmacol Bull 1992;28(1):61-66.

14. Monteleone P, et al. Effects of phosphatidylserine on the neuroendocrine response to physical stress in humans. Neuroendocrinology 1990 Sep;52(3):243-8.

15. Monteleone P, et al. Blunting by chronic phosphatidylserine administration of the stress-induced activation of the hypothalamo-pituitary-adrenal axis in healthy men. Eur J Clin Pharmacol 1992;42(4):385-388.

16. Benton D, et al. The influence of phosphatidylserine supplementation on mood and heart rate when faced with an acute stressor. Nutr Neurosci 2001;4(3):169-78.

17. Ross J. Eliminating the top causes of insomnia: neurotransmitter deficiency and cortisol excess. The Townsend Letter, October 2011.

18. Hirayama S, Terasawa K et al. The effect of phosphatidylserine administration on memory and symptoms of attention-deficit hyperactivity disorder: a randomised, double-blind, placebo-controlled clinical trial. J Hum Nutr Diet. 2014 Apr;27 Suppl 2:284-91.

Taurine

1. Murakami S. Taurine and atherosclerosis. Amino Acids. 2014 Jan;46(1):73-80.

2. Azuma J, Sawamura A et al. Therapeutic effect of

taurine in congestive heart failure: a double-blind crossover trial. Clin Cardiol. 1985 May;8(5):276-82.

3. Gebara E, Udry F et al. Taurine increases hippocampal neurogenesis in aging mice. Stem Cell Res. 2015 May;14 (3):369-79.

4. Pasantes-Morales H, Ramos-Mandujano G et al. Taurine enhances proliferation and promotes neuronal specification of murine and human neural stem/progenitor cells. Adv Exp Med Biol. 2015;803:457-72.

5. Liu J, Wang HW et al. Antenatal taurine improves neuronal regeneration in fetal rats with intrauterine growth restriction by inhibiting the Rho-ROCK signal pathway. Metab Brain Dis. 2015 Feb;30(1):67-73.

6. Hernández-Benítez R, Vangipuram SD, et al. Taurine enhances the growth of neural precursors derived from fetal human brain and promotes neuronal specification. Dev Neurosci. 2013;35(1):40-9.

7. Gebara E, Udry F et al. Taurine increases hippocampal neurogenesis in aging mice. Stem Cell Res. 2015 May;14 (3):369-79.

8. Toyoda A, Koike H et al. Effects of chronic taurine administration on gene expression, protein translation and phosphorylation in the rat hippocampus. Adv Exp Med Biol. 2015;803:473-80.

9. Ferguson CA, Audesirk G. Effects of DDT and permethrin on neurite growth in cultured neurons of chick embryo brain and Lymnaea stagnalis. Toxicol In Vitro. 1990;4 (1):23-30.

10. Chou C, Lin H et al. Taurine resumed neuronal differentiation in arsenite-treated N2a cells through reducing oxidative stress, endoplasmic reticulum stress, and mitochon-

drial dysfunction. Amino Acids. 2015 Apr;47(4):735-44.

11. Montanini R et al: Taurine in the management of diffuse cerebral arteriopathy. Clinical and electroencephalographic observations, and mental test results. Clin Ter 71 (5):427-36, 1974.

12. Ikeda H. Effects of taurine on alcohol withdrawal. Lancet 1977;2:509.

13. Zhang L, Yuan Y et al. Reduced plasma taurine level in Parkinson's disease: association with motor severity and levodopa treatment. Int J Neurosci. 2015 May 23:1-24.

14. Liu HY, Gao WY et al. Taurine modulates calcium influx through L-type voltage-gated calcium channels in isolated cochlear outer hair cells in guinea pigs. Neurosci Lett. 2006 May 15;399(1-2):23-6.

15. Liu HY, Chi FL et al. Taurine modulates calcium influx under normal and ototoxic conditions in isolated cochlear spiral ganglion neurons. Pharmacol Rep. 2008b Jul-Aug;60 (4):508-13.

16. Brozoski TJ, Caspary DM et al. The effect of supplemental dietary taurine on tinnitus and auditory discrimination in an animal model. Hear Res. 2010 Dec 1;270(1-2):71-80.

17. Allen MJ. Successful Reversal of Retinitis Pigmentosa. Journal of Orthomolecular Medicine, 1998;13(1):41-43. Indiana University School of Optometry, Bloomington, Indiana, USA.

18. Rea W. Chemical Sensitivity Volume 1. Lewis Publishers, Boca Raton, USA, 1992.

19. Watanabe A, Hobara N, Nagashima H. Lowering of Liver Acetaldehyde but Not Ethanol Concentrations by Pretreatment With Taurine in Ethanol-Loaded Rats. Experien-

tia, 1985;41:1421-422.
20. Rosa F, Freitas E et al. Oxidative stress and inflammation in obesity after taurine supplementation: a double-blind, placebo-controlled study. Eur J Nutr. 2014 Apr;53(3):823-30.
21. Franconi F, Bennardini F, Mattana A, et al. Plasma and platelet taurine are reduced in subjects with insulin-dependent diabetes mellitus: effects of taurine supplementation. Am J Clin Nutr. 1995 May;61(5):1115-9.
22. Chen W, Guo J et al. The beneficial effects of taurine in preventing metabolic syndrome. Food Funct. 2016 Apr 20;7(4):1849-63] [De la Puerta C, Arrieta FJ et al. Taurine and glucose metabolism: a review. Nutr Hosp. 2010 Nov-Dec;25(6):910-9.
23. Das J, Roy A, Sil PC. Mechanism of the protective action of taurine in toxin and drug induced organ pathophysiology and diabetic complications: a review. Food Funct. 2012;3(12):1251–64.
24. Carrasco S, Codoceo R et al. Department of Pediatrics, Children's Hospital La Paz, Autonoma University, Madrid, Spain. Effect of taurine supplements on growth, fat absorption and bile acid on cystic fibrosis. Acta Univ Carol [Med] (Praha) 1990;36(1-4):152-6.
25. Shao A, Hathcock JN. Risk assessment for the amino acids taurine, L-glutamine and L-arginine. Regul Toxicol Pharmacol. 2008 Apr;50(3):376-99.

Threonine

1. Braverman ER. The Healing Nutrients Within. Keats Publishing Inc., New Canaan, USA, 1997.
2. Barbeau A, Roy M, Chouza C. Pilot study of threonine

supplementation in human spasticity. Canadian Journal of Neurological Science 1982 May;9(2):141-5.

3. Lee K-C et al. The Antispastic Effect of L-Threonine. Amino Acids, Chemistry, Biology and Medicine, 1990;658-663. Department of Neurology, Royal Victoria Hospital, Belfast, Northern Ireland.

4. Hauser SL et al. Antispasticity Effect of Threonine in Multiple Sclerosis. Archives of Neurology, September 1992;49:923-926. Neuroimmunology Unit, Massachusetts General Hospital, Boston, Massachusetts, USA.

5. Rude RK, Singer FR, Gruber HE. Skeletal and hormonal effects of magnesium deficiency. J Am Coll Nutr. 2009 Apr;28(2):131-41.

6. Slutsky I, Abumaria N, Wu LJ, et al. Enhancement of learning and memory by elevating brain magnesium. Neuron. 2010 Jan 28;65(2):165-77.

Tryptophan

1. Payton A, Gibbons L, Davidson Y, et al. Influence of serotonin transporter gene polymorphisms on cognitive decline and cognitive abilities in a nondemented elderly population. Mol Psychiatry. 2005 Dec;10(12):1133-9.

2. Murray MF, Langan M, MacGregor RR. Increased plasma tryptophan in HIV-infected patients treated with pharmacologic doses of nicotinamide. Nutrition. 2001 Jul;17(7-8):654-6.

3. Castell LM, Yamamoto T et al. University Department of Biochemistry, Oxford, UK. The role of tryptophan in fatigue in different conditions of stress. Adv Exp Med Biol 1999;467:697-704.

4. Hoshino Y, Yamamoto T, Kaneko M, et al. Blood Sero-

tonin and Free Tryptophan Concentration in Autistic Children. Neuropsychobiology, 1984;11:22-27.

5. Patrick RP, Ames BN. Vitamin D hormone regulates serotonin synthesis. Part 1: relevance for autism. FASEB J. 2014 Jun;28(6):2398-413.

6. Toker L, Amar S, Bersudsky Y, Benjamin J, Klein E. The biology of tryptophan depletion and mood disorders. Isr J Psychiatry Relat Sci. 2010;47(1):46-55.

7. Ruhé HG, Mason NS, Schene AH. Mood is indirectly related to serotonin, norepinephrine and dopamine levels in humans: a meta-analysis of monoamine depletion studies. Mol Psychiatry. 2007 Apr;12(4):331-59.

8. Braverman ER. The Healing Nutrients Within. Keats Publishing Inc., New Canaan, USA, 1997.

9. Ghadirian AM, Murphy BE, et al. Efficacy of light versus tryptophan therapy in seasonal affective disorder. J Affect Disord. 1998;50(1):23–7.

10. Jangid P, Malik P at al. Comparative study of efficacy of l-5-hydroxytryptophan and fluoxetine in patients presenting with first depressive episode. Asian J Psychiatr. 2013 Feb;6(1):29-34.

11. Rea W. Chemical Sensitivity Volume I. Lewis Publishers, Boca Raton, USA, 1992.

12. Robinson OJ, Overstreet C et al. Acute tryptophan depletion increases translational indices of anxiety but not fear: serotonergic modulation of the bed nucleus of the stria terminalis? Neuropsychopharmacology. 2012 Jul;37(8):1963-71.

13. Cleare AJ, Bond AJ. The Effect of Tryptophan Depletion and Enhancement on Subjective and Behavioural Aggression in Normal Male Subjects. Psychopharmacology,

1995;118:72-81.

14. Volavka J, Crowner M, Brizer D, et al. Tryptophan Treatment of Aggressive Psychiatric Inpatients. Biol Psychiatry, October 15, 1990;28(8):728-732.

15. Katting WF, Bubenzer S et al. Effects of tryptophan depletion on reactive aggression and aggressive decision-making in young people with ADHD. Acta Psychiatr Scand. 2013 Aug;128(2):114-23.

16. McCloskey MS, Ben-Zeev D et al. Acute tryptophan depletion and self-injurious behavior in aggressive patients and healthy volunteers. Psychopharmacology (Berl). 2009 Mar;203(1):53-61.

17. Aan het Rot M, Moskowitz DS et al. Social behaviour and mood in everyday life: the effects of tryptophan in quarrelsome individuals. J Psychiatry Neurosci. 2006 Jul;31(4):253-62.

18. Bond AJ, Wingrove J et al. Tryptophan depletion increases aggression in women during the premenstrual phase. Psychopharmacology (Berl). 2001 Aug;156(4):477-80.

19. Walderhaug E, Lunde H et al. Lowering of serotonin by rapid tryptophan depletion increases impulsiveness in normal individuals. Psychopharmacology (Berl). 2002 Dec;164(4):385-91.

20. Westrick ER, Shapiro AP, Nathan PE, Brick J. Alcohol Behavior Research Laboratory, Rutgers State University of New Jersey, Piscataway, USA. Dietary tryptophan reverses alcohol-induced impairment of facial recognition but not verbal recall. Alcohol Clin Exp Res 1988 Aug;12(4):531-3.

21. Pihl RO et al. Acute effect of altered tryptophan levels and alcohol on aggression in normal human males. Psy-

chopharmacology. 1995;119(4):353-60.
22. Asheychik R, Jackson T, Baker H, et al. The efficacy of L-tryptophan in the reduction of sleep disturbance and depressive state in alcoholic patients. J Stud Alcohol. 1989 Nov;50(6):525-32.
23. Sandyk R, Fisher H. Department of Neurology, University of Arizona, Tucson, USA. L-tryptophan supplementation in Parkinson's disease. International Journal of Neuroscience 1989 Apr;45(3-4):215-9.
24. Sandyk R. L-tryptophan in Neuropsychiatric disorders: a review. Int J Neurosci. 1992 Nov- Dec;67(1-4):127-44.
25. Capitelli C, Sereniki A et al. Melatonin attenuates tyrosine hydroxylase loss and hypolocomotion in MPTP-lesioned rats. Eur J Pharmacol. 2008 Oct 10;594(1-3):101-8.
26. Klongpanichapak S, Phansuwan-Pujito P et al. Melatonin inhibits amphetamine-induced increase in alpha-synuclein and decrease in phosphorylated tyrosine hydroxylase in SK-N-SH cells. Neurosci Lett. 2008 May 16;436(3):309-13.
27. Sandyk R. NeuroCommunication Research Laboratories, Danbury, CT 06811, USA. Tryptophan availability and the susceptibility to stress in multiple sclerosis: a hypothesis. International Journal of Neuroscience 1996 Jul;86 (1-2):47-53.
28. Haze JJ. Newark Beth Israel Medical Center, USA. Toward an understanding of the rationale for the use of dietary supplementation for chronic pain management: the serotonin model. Craniology 1991 Oct;9(4):339-43.
29. Segura R, Ventura JL. Department of Physiological Sciences and Nutrition, Medical School, University of Bar-

celona, Spain. Effect of L-tryptophan supplementation on exercise performance. International Journal of Sports Medicine 1988 Oct;9(5):301-5.

30. Javierre C, Segura R et al. L-tryptophan supplementation can decrease fatigue perception during an aerobic exercise with supramaximal intercalated anaerobic bouts in young healthy men. Int J Neurosci. 2010 May;120(5):319-27.

31. Cangiano C, Ceci F, Cascino A et al. Eating behavior and adherence to dietary prescriptions in obese adult subjects treated with 5-hydroxytryptophan. Am J Clin Nutr 1992 Nov;56(5):863-7. 3rd Department of Internal Medicine, University of Rome, Italy.

32. Gendall KA, Joyce PR. Meal-induced changes in tryptophan:LNAA ratio: effects on craving and binge eating. Eat Behav. 2000 Sep;1(1):53-62.

33. Cavaliere H, Medeiros-Neto G. The anorectic effect of increasing doses of L-tryptophan in obese patients. Eat Weight Disord. 1997 Dec;2(4):211-5.

34. Sarzi Puttini P et al. Primary fibromyalgia syndrome and 5-hydroxy-L-tryptophan: a 90-day open study. J Int Med Res. 1992 Apr;20(2):182-9.

35. Steinberg S, Annable L, Young SN, Liyanage N. A placebo-controlled clinical trial of L-tryptophan in premenstrual dysphoria. Biol Psychiatry. 1999 Feb 1;45(3):313-20.

36. Haspels AA, Bennink HJ, Schreurs WH. Disturbance of tryptophan metabolism and its correction during oestrogen treatment in postmenopausal women. Maturitas 1978 Jun;1(1):15-20.

37. Hudson C, Hudson SP, Hecht T, MacKenzie J. Protein source tryptophan versus pharmaceutical grade tryptophan

as an efficacious treatment for chronic insomnia. Nutr Neurosci. 2005 Apr;8(2):121-7.

38. Hartmann E, Spinweber CL. Sleep induced by L-tryptophan. Effect of dosages within the normal dietary intake. J Nerv Ment.Dis. 1979 Aug;167(8):497-9.

39. Lieberman HR, Corkin S et al. The effects of dietary neurotransmitter precursors on human behavior. Am J Clin Nutr. 1985 Aug;42(2):366-70.

40. Raleigh MJ. Differential Behavioral Effects of Tryptophan and 5-Hydroxytryptophan in Vervet Monkeys: Influence of Catecholaminergic Systems. Psychopharmacology 1987;93:44-50.

Tyrosine

1. Møller SE, Maach-Møller B et al. Tyrosine metabolism in users of oral contraceptives. Life Sci. 1995;56(9):687-95

2. Lemoine P, Robelin N, Sebert P, Mouret J. Unite clinique de Psychiatrie biologique, C.H.S. Le Vinatier, Lyon-Bron. [L-tyrosine: a long term treatment of Parkinson's disease]. [Article in French] C R Acad Sci III 1989;309(2):43-7.

3. Siniscalchi A, Mancuso F et al. Increase in plasma homocysteine levels induced by drug treatments in neurologic patients. Pharmacol Res. 2005 Nov;52(5):367-75.

4. Tan EK, Cheah SY, Fook-Chong S, et al. Functional COMT variant predicts response to high dose pyridoxine in Parkinson's disease. Am J Med Genet B Neuropsychiatr Genet. 2005 Aug 5;137B(1):1-4.

5. Amadasi A, Bertoldi M, Contestabile R, et al. Pyridoxal 5'-phosphate enzymes as targets for therapeutic agents. Curr Med Chem. 2007;14(12):1291-324.

6. Evatt ML, Delong MR et al. Prevalence of vitamin D insufficiency in patients with Parkinson disease and Alzheimer disease. Arch Neurol. 2008 Oct;65(10):1348-52.

7. Cui X, Pertile R, Liu P, Eyles DW. Vitamin D regulates tyrosine hydroxylase expression: N-cadherin a possible mediator. Neuroscience. 2015 Sep 24;304:90-100.

8. Cho HS, Kim S et al. Protective effect of the green tea component, L-theanine on environmental toxins-induced neuronal cell death. Neurotoxicology. 2008 Jul;29(4):656-62.

9. Mandel SA, Amit T et al. Simultaneous manipulation of multiple brain targets by green tea catechins: a potential neuroprotective strategy for Alzheimer and Parkinson diseases. CNS Neurosci Ther. 2008 Winter;14(4):352-65.

10. Zhao B. Natural antioxidants protect neurons in Alzheimer's disease and Parkinson's disease. Neurochem Res. 2009 Apr;34(4):630-8.

11. Snider SR. Octacosanol in parkinsonism. (Letter). Annals of Neurology 16(6):723, 1984.

12. Neri DF, Wiegmann D et al. Naval Aerospace Medical Research Laboratory, Pensacola, USA. The effects of tyrosine on cognitive performance during extended wakefulness. Aviat Space Environ Med. 1995 Apr;66(4):313-9.

13. Owasoyo JO, et al. Tyrosine and its potential use as a countermeasure to performance decrement in military sustained operations. Aviation, Space, and Environmental Medicine, May 1992;364-369.

14. Tumilty L, Davison G et al. Oral tyrosine supplementation improves exercise capacity in the heat. Eur J Appl Physiol. 2011 Dec;111(12):2941-50.

15. Mahoney CR, Castellani J et al. Tyrosine supplementa-

tion mitigates working memory decrements during cold exposure. Physiol Behav. 2007 Nov 23;92(4):575-82.

16. Deijen JB, Orlebeke JF. Effect of tyrosine on cognitive function and blood pressure under stress. Brain Res Bull. 1994;33(3):319-23.

17. Deijen JB, Wientjes CJ et al. Department of Clinical Neuropsychology, Vrije Universiteit, Amsterdam, The Netherlands. Tyrosine improves cognitive performance and reduces blood pressure in cadets after one week of a combat training course. Brain Research Bulletin 1999 Jan 15;48 (2):203-9.

18. Steenbergen L, Sellaro R et al. Tyrosine promotes cognitive flexibility: evidence from proactive vs. reactive control during task switching performance. Neuropsychologia. 2015 Mar;69:50-5.

19. Thomas JR, Lockwood PA et al. Department of Military and Emergency Medicine, Bethesda, USA. Tyrosine improves working memory in a multitasking environment. Pharmacol Biochem Behav. 1999 Nov;64(3):495-500.

20. Braverman ER. The Healing Nutrients Within. Keats Publishing Inc., New Canaan, USA, 1997.

21. Mouret J et al: L-tyrosine cures, immediate and long term, dopamine-dependent depressions. Clinical and polygraphic studies (in French). C R Acad Sci III 306(3):9308, 1988.

22. Gelenberg AJ et al: Tyrosine for depression. J Psychiatr Res 17(2):175-80, 1982.

23. Goldberg IK. L-Tyrosine in Depression. Lancet, August 16, 1980:364.

24. Rose DP, Cramp DG. Reduction of Plasma Tyrosine by Oral Contraceptives and Oestrogens: A Possible Conse-

quence of Tyrosine Aminotransferase Induction. Clin Chim Acta, 1970;29:49-53.

Valine

1. Castell LM, Yamamoto T et al. University Department of Biochemistry, Oxford, UK. The role of tryptophan in fatigue in different conditions of stress. Adv Exp Med Biol 1999;467:697-704.

INDEX

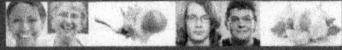

The School of Modern Naturopathy

Have you ever thought about training as a naturopathic nutritionist? This is a natural health consultant who specializes in creating tailored health programs which can help individuals overcome common health problems and ailments.

Linda Lazarides teaches a one-year diploma course by distance learning, using a combination of specially written course modules and internet-based teaching. This course is accredited by major organizations in the United Kingdom, United States, Australia and New Zealand. Graduates are also eligible to practice in Canada. Upon successful completion, you would be qualified to work as a wellness counsellor, health coach, naturopathic nutritionist or nutrition advisor. You would be eligible to set up in private practice, or work in a health club, health food store or perhaps for a vitamin or natural products company.

If you plan to work as a writer or journalist, you would gain an in-depth understanding of holistic health which would greatly improve the quality of your books and articles and also make it much easier for you to find ideas and reliable information for articles to interest your readers.

Linda Lazarides is a master practitioner and founder of the British Association for Nutritional Therapy. In 1996 she helped the University of Westminster to set up the UK's first degree course in Nutritional Therapy. and previously for several years worked as a complementary practitioner for the British National Health Service. She has been a nutrition editor for the International Journal of Alternative and Complementary Medicine, an advisor to several national organizations, and has been invited to speak at parliamentary committees in the UK.

For more information about the School of Modern Naturopathy, and to read the course prospectus, please visit www.naturostudy.org.

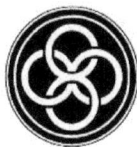

International Institute for
Complementary Therapists
IICT APPROVED
TRAINING PROVIDER

Easy Water Retention Diet

by Linda Lazarides

Water retention looks like fat and makes you overweight. But you can't lose it by eating less.

Many thousands of people fail to lose weight on a normal, low-calorie diet. This is usually because of hormonal problems (which can be diagnosed by your doctor) or because of water retention.

Until recently, there was no medical treatment for water retention, except diuretics, which have only a temporary effect and can worsen some types of water retention.

Linda Lazarides' water retention diet is a new treatment. It targets seven different types of water retention and makes your kidneys (if they are normal and healthy) release the excess fluid.

You can literally urinate away pounds of your excess body weight

- Have you worked hard to lose weight using conventional methods, and found that you cannot get below a certain weight even if you persevere for months or years?
- Do your ankles ever swell up? Does your shoe size seem to increase as you get older? Do your rings sometimes seem not to fit you any more? Is your tummy often tight and swollen?
- If you are a woman, do you often suffer from breast tenderness?
- Does your weight ever fluctuate by several pounds within the space of only 24 hours?

If you can answer yes to two or more of these questions you may have hidden water retention

The *Easy Water Retention Diet* explains why water tablets and diuretics don't work for idiopathic edema (the most common type of water retention) and could actually make it worse. The book explains the causes of water retention and provides a one-week program offering a significant reduction in idiopathic edema for up to 70 per cent of those who follow the diet.

Available from Amazon websites and all good bookshops

Ask for ISBN 978-1519191472

A Textbook of
Modern Naturopathy

by Linda Lazarides

Covers a wide variety of important lecture topics in the naturopathic or natural medicine curriculum. These are topics that every student of holistic health needs to know, including information rarely covered elsewhere: healthy infant nutrition, kidney health, fertility, the microcirculation, the nervous system, metabolic sediment, cell membrane health, the effects of deep-fried foods, moulds (molds) and mycotoxins, and Ayurvedic principles.

Apart from aiming to complement the many excellent publications which are already used as course-books, the author hopes that *A Textbook of Modern Naturopathy* will also play a holistic teaching role—helping to bridge some of the gaps in understanding disease processes and helping the student practitioner to see each problem and each research study in relation to the bigger picture.

Reviews

'This is the most complete book I have found on natural health and healing.'

'I was so impressed that I have chosen her course to train as a naturopath.'

'Very well written book leading one to understand the fundamentals of naturopathy.'

'I found much of her input on subjects such as the management of supporting HIV or chronic dysbiosis interesting and provocative.'

'Best natural healing book I've found so far .'

'Every chapter of this book is well written and easy to read. A tremendous amount of useful information is packed into each chapter. It is one of my favorite books.'

Rated 5 stars on goodreads.com and amazon.co.uk

Look for the *Textbook of Modern Naturopathy* online, or order ISBN 978-1450549929 from bookstores

Lightning Source UK Ltd.
Milton Keynes UK
UKHW022022050520
362826UK00013B/219

9 781533 377326